W0038431

"Beyond the clinical intricacies, Bentley introduces the reader to a diverse cast of healthcare providers—from medics to nurses to intensivists—shedding light on their roles and underscoring the profound significance of compassionate care. The relationships that serve as lifelines during this tumultuous journey are meticulously examined, encompassing family, friends, medical staff, and the solace found in faith.

"John Bentley's unique position, grappling with the storm and enduring the devastating loss of a child, offers a perspective seldom experienced in twenty-first-century America. Through his narrative, he crafts a compelling and emotionally charged account that resonates with the honesty and raw courage required to navigate such profound grief. *Katie Girl* emerges as an offering of potential solace and insight to those grappling with insurmountable loss and stands as a valuable addition to curricula in medical training, providing crucial insights for healthcare providers engaged in the care of critically ill patients."

—Geoff Fitzgerald, MD, FACEP

"*Katie Girl* is an unflinching account of a family's loss of their four-year-old daughter to sudden illness, and a tribute to all those who work in the healthcare field. It is also a testimony to the unpredictable moments of grace that follow in tragedy's wake. A lifelong resident of rural New Hampshire, John Bentley has written a Yankee memoir of grief, delivered in a matter-of-fact style, and shorn of sentimentality. And yet throughout his story, the author bears witness to the everyday kindness of ordinary heroes, as well as to the extraordinary intimations he glimpsed of an unseen world beyond our own. This book is both a heartbreaking tale, lovingly recounted, and a sustained spiritual reflection on bereavement and death."

—Darryl Caterine, PhD, Professor of
Religious Studies, Le Moyne College

"*Katie Girl* is a powerful story of one family's experience of terrible loss, simply and honestly told. While Katie Bentley's illness was rare enough to draw national attention, the story is universal. All of us lose those we love, in spite of the best efforts of our doctors and nurses. This book captures the dashed hopes, fear, and grief of losing a child, and serves as a testimony to the skilled and compassionate men and women who work in our hospitals. And ultimately, this story shows how the bereaved parents, supported by each other, their family, and their community, found a way to move forward with their lives."

—Ernest Freeberg, PhD, Distinguished Professor of
Humanities, University of Tennessee-Knoxville

"In *Katie Girl*, first-time author John Bentley, of, Salisbury, New Hampshire, finds himself (and his wife and family) face-to-face with every parent's most dreaded nightmare: the diagnosis of a child with a life-threatening illness. In four-year-old Katie's case, the illness is both exceedingly rare and perplexingly incurable.

"The reader will be enriched beyond measure to consider how the story of Katie Girl and her parents offers inspiration, how perhaps we can partake of the grace offered in their story, to transform our own personal tragedies into 'little' triumphs, and where necessary, even to change ourselves."

—D. Stephen Cloniger, MDiv, PhD, Huntersville, North Carolina

"*Katie Girl* is an important story on a hundred fronts. Important as a record, as a tribute, as a history, as a monument. But most of all, it sets the mind to focus on what is important and what a slender thread our joy hangs by. Katie's story helps us to begin to understand the gift that life is and how briefly we own happiness."

—Roger Heath, Educator and Former New Hampshire State Senator

Advance Readers' Comments for *Katie Girl*

"*Katie Girl* by John S. Bentley is an incredibly important and powerful book describing the unthinkable tragedy of losing his previously healthy four-year-old daughter to a rare and aggressive infection despite every intervention modern medicine has to offer. This is an absolute must-read to all healthcare providers and parents alike!

"Losing a child is often a taboo subject in our society and not many people want to or can talk or even ask about it. John's beautiful writing, his openness, honesty, vulnerability, and courage make it not only possible but heart-warming and enormously enriching to go there. Instead of a tearjerker story that might be difficult to read, as a reader you accompany John on his journey how events unfolded, the details of what his family went through, the medical facts, how people were touched by Katie's life and death, and her incredible legacy to the world. John describes the lows but also the highs of a tragedy like this—full of love and hope, humility and respect, joy and pain, gratitude and criticism.

"I happened to have the privilege of taking care of Katie briefly during her illness and meeting John during my training as a pediatric intensive care physician. I was very early in my training at the time and was learning so many things from her that one night that I will be forever grateful for. Reading John's book taught me even more.

"As physicians, we often do not have the opportunity to fully get to know our patients or their families, understand their perspective, or get more than a glimpse of what they are truly going through. This book allows a deep dive into Katie's family's life and experiences, especially during their most difficult and challenging times, and to witness their amazing strength, hope, and capacity to heal. It is the ultimate gift that John through Katie's story is giving his readers.

"Through learning about the love, hope, and support for Katie and her family, witnessing how people and community can come together to lift each other up and support a grieving family through the worst nightmare for any parent, I came to an understanding, inspiration, and awe that would forever be unknown to me and probably would be to the reader, too, had John not written this book. Katie's life, as full of joy and love as it was, was much too short; but her legacy will live on forever (not only in this book!) and is beyond humbling and inspiring."

—Stefanie Gauguet, MD, PhD, Pediatric Intensive Care Physician

"Health care workers will learn the emotional intricacies of families with seriously ill family members and how best to support them. All families who have ever experienced the unexpected death of a family member, particularly a child, will learn valuable lessons about the medical system and the emotional journey involved. Even news media can learn a few things. And the rest of us learn how to support others when tragedy hits.

"John Bentley, a plain-speaking, plain-living, but well-educated man who knows how to tell a good story, invites us into the most intimate moments of his family's life during the illness and death of their four-year-old daughter, and the family's difficult journey of coping and recovery. You will cry, but you will be inspired, educated, and uplifted too. And you might even learn why lilacs should be your favorite flower."

—Mark L. DeBard, MD, FACEP, Professor Emeritus of Clinical
    Emergency Medicine, The Ohio State University College of Medicine

"In *Katie Girl*, John Bentley candidly shares his journey as a parent thrust into the daunting realm of caring for a once healthy child suddenly confronted by a life-threatening illness. Bentley's down-to-earth, common-sense approach narrative style peels back the layers of medical procedures and technology. As his family navigates through the corridors of a community hospital and a tertiary care ICU, the author describes in lay terms the intricate web of our modern healthcare systems technologies and procedures.

"Katie Bentley was a young girl so full of life. I remember the first day I met her. I would be taking care of her while John and Cheryl worked. John dropped her off at my house in Salisbury, New Hampshire, and left for work for the day. She was just a baby then. When Cheryl came to pick her up later that day, she found Katie asleep in my arms, with her head on my shoulder. She was in shock. 'How did you do that? She won't do that with us, she just doesn't like to sleep.' And from then on, Katie grew into the rambunctious, fun-loving, beautiful child written about in this book. She didn't want to miss a thing.

"Here John writes the story of Katie, the amazing doctors, nurses, and caregivers who helped them through this terrible ordeal and of the community coming together in a time of crisis. The medical detail provided comes from the patience and kindness of the medical staff at both hospitals, realizing that they had a family trying to cope with the reality of a critically ill child. They realized that they not only had Katie as a patient, but the whole family. They had to make decisions quickly, but also keep John and Cheryl informed in a way non-medical personnel could comprehend. It's also a story about faith and family surviving a tragedy and handling the cards they were dealt with grace. They not only survived, but through this book are trying to help other families and medical professionals deal with and learn from circumstances such as theirs."

—Sue Linares, Caregiver, Paramedic

Katie Girl

by
John S. Bentley

ISBN: 978-1-942155-78-2
Library of Congress Control No. 2024912387

Published by
Peter E. Randall Publisher
5 Greenleaf Woods Drive, #102
Portsmouth, NH, 03801
www.perpublisher.com

Book Design: Tim Holtz

Contents

Foreword

This unassuming yet profound book is a mirror. For families, it begins as an almost casual conversation, relating events as one parent might share experiences with another. At the start, most would be familiar with the situations and nod in agreement: been there, done that. But as the story unfolds, the ordinary is shattered, and we share mounting terror as the reflection of everyday life becomes one of a lightning strike and a new reality.

When events unfold down an unimaginable, out-of-control path, the story becomes a mirror for those of us in the medical profession. Mr. Bentley accurately presents technical information from a layman's perspective and, in doing so, helps us understand what we look like, what we are charged with, and what happens when we fail. Every medical student, resident, fellow, nurse, and attending physician can read this, see themselves, and aspire to be better. For pediatricians in particular, it is a rare opportunity to see our reflection in the eyes of an unusually articulate and discerning parent.

In the aftermath of the medical events, *Katie Girl* becomes a mirror of our society. The stark reminder of human fragility in a frightening and uncertain world brings responses ranging from media hype to pure and humble altruism. As we witness this full range of behavior, we are reminded that our response is our own choice, those choices have consequences, and the world we live in is what we make it.

Finally, for those of us who have experienced loss, this remarkable book offers a poignant reflection of our despair and helplessness. Yet in that reflection, we can begin to glimpse elements in the background, things behind and all around us, that may not be visible directly. We come to see that there are personal, spiritual, and metaphysical aspects of our world from which we can draw the courage and meaning necessary to carry on.

For many of us, the Bentley family journey is our journey and a reflection of our best selves as we try to navigate it. For all of us, it is an invitation to see ourselves, others, and our larger society through a lens of empathy, insight, and hope.

Michael L. McManus, MD, MPH

Preface

People ask me why I wrote this book. I never have a good answer. I never thought about why, I just did it. It started as a chronicle of events during my daughter Katie's hospitalization. I wanted a record of what happened, for us, for Katie when she got better and came home, and for other family members. The information coming at us was overpowering and exhausting. We didn't understand it and we couldn't keep track of it. I started keeping a journal every evening after we left Katie's bedside, jotting down notes on the laptop as I remembered them, trying to make sense of it all. There were new words, new terms, and new concepts delivered to us every day, all of it delivered in an atmosphere of confusion, bewilderment, worry, and terror. We had no idea what was happening, none of it made any sense; we struggled to absorb it.

One of Katie's doctors said to me years later that she couldn't believe how calm I was on the first night. Soon she realized that I was clueless about what was really happening, so the medical team had to take a different approach with me, as a secondary patient. They translated the language from medical into layman's terms, and kept asking me if I knew what it meant, without revealing their own fears. They didn't want me to have a mental breakdown; that would have to wait for later.

I started writing this book five months after the events with Katie. I kept notes in the hospital every day, so I had something to start with for an outline. I worked on it after supper, when we had put our daughter Molly to bed and the house was quiet. I was able to create the framework in eight days, but it took years to put the finishing touches on it. Originally, it was supposed to be a brief chronicle for the family archives, so that family members would have a record of what happened. Though they lived through it with us, there were a lot of questions left unanswered, a lot of details that were never told. When it happened, neither my wife, Cheryl, nor I could discern a path forward. We took things one day at a time and dealt with it head on, together. The shock was profound and induced silence, from us and everyone else. The written word would help to explain that which conversation would not allow.

I didn't understand most of the medical terminology that we learned, so as the storyline progressed, I would send it to some of Katie's doctors in Boston to review the technical and medical details, hoping to get it right. After several of these email exchanges, one of her doctors suggested that it was more than just a family record, that it could be helpful to other parents in similar situations, and also to the medical community. He encouraged me to publish it.

I sought advice from my friends in academia, all published authors, several of whom edited it for me, and offered suggestions about the timeline and other details. I went over it and over it, chopping out whole sections and expanding others. I remember watching a documentary on Mark Twain's writing, and I recall the researcher showing working proofs of Twain's books. The narrator commented that Twain didn't get everything right the first time. His words were, "He had to chisel it out." That's what it felt like.

Sometimes it lay fallow for an entire year while I battled other problems and raised our two girls. One of my friends put me in touch with a professional editor in New York City, who agreed to take it. His work was important in turning it into a readable story. Much of the detail of the trouble with the newspaper and television reporters I discarded, on his advice. Though their behavior was invasive and incomprehensible, it distracted from the storyline. The support we received from hundreds of others is what the story is really about, an invigorating salutation to humanity. It is also a tale of how two ordinary, average people faced the unthinkable, worked through it, survived the ordeal, and were eventually able to return to a degree of normalcy; some support groups refer to it as the "New Normal."

What follows is the cumulative effort of many people, all of whom had a role in creating the finished product. I am grateful for their interest and support in bringing the story to you.

CHAPTER 1

Imminent Obscurity

As the helicopter lifted off the helipad, the lights of our local hospital in Concord, New Hampshire, grew fainter and the building appeared to shrink in size. As I watched out the window, it looked like things were moving away from me, not that I was moving away from them. I had no sensation of flying, only of movement, accompanied by a robust shaking. I hate helicopters. This one felt like it was going to shake itself apart and send me crashing to the ground in a hail of torn aluminum and shattered rotors. But this Saturday night, now eleven o'clock, we made it into the dark New Hampshire sky and headed toward Boston, Massachusetts, with my four-year-old little Katie girl strapped to a gurney beside me and a flight nurse monitoring her vital signs.

I didn't know it at the time, but Katie's school nurse, who lives just one block away from the hospital, had heard the chopper coming in for a landing. She always says a prayer for the person who is going out on the helicopter. She saw that it was headed south, which was unusual. Normally it would go north, toward the large hospital in Lebanon, New Hampshire. She commented to her husband, "I hope that isn't one of my students." She had an eerie, inexplicable feeling that it might be, though not because Katie had been sick at school or visited the nurse's office. The nurse said another prayer as the chopper droned out of hearing range.

Only three and a half hours earlier, at seven thirty, Katie had walked with me into the emergency department with a fever and a cough. Now we were headed for a bigger hospital, one with more resources to deal with a very sick child. The helicopter, a Kawasaki MBB/BK117C1, was one of the most popular air ambulance helicopter models in the world. We were traveling at 120 miles per hour at an altitude of two thousand feet as we approached the city lights of Boston. In 1858, Oliver Wendell Holmes declared that Boston was the Hub of the Universe. I was soon to learn that nickname, when applied to medicine, was close to the mark.

As we flew over Boston at low altitude the Citgo sign at Fenway Park was clearly visible, though so small that I thought at first it must be just a large filling station. The Citgo sign is the largest sign in New England, measuring sixty feet wide by sixty feet high, the length of a tractor trailer and the height of a six-story building. It's hard to miss. It was only when we passed directly over the baseball field and started to descend that I realized it was the big sign at the back of the field. Twenty-seven minutes and fifty-six air miles later, we landed on the roof of our destination, the best pediatric hospital in the United States, at eleven thirty.

Katie was a strong four-year-old girl. During the week she went to preschool in the morning, and to daycare in the afternoon, where she could play with her two-year-old sister, Molly. Yesterday, Friday, she had gone to both, with no symptoms of sickness.

We live in Salisbury, New Hampshire, a small town northwest of the state capital, Concord. I was born there, and my family has been here for four generations. I am a self-employed contractor, a job I decided to do after spending too many years in higher education as a lower-level administrator. I set my own hours, so I always dropped off and picked up the girls by myself at daycare or preschool, due to my wife Cheryl's work schedule. She worked for a US government agency as a federal wildlife biologist. But yesterday, Cheryl was sick, and stayed home from work. She had a cold that she had acquired from Molly a few days earlier, so she was able to go with me to get them. We were not greatly surprised when we found that Katie felt out of sorts and appeared to be getting the same cold. The kids would often catch a cold from their classmates, and bring it home to share with the family.

Cheryl took Katie's temperature when we got home and found it to be elevated, at 100.5 degrees. She gave her some children's ibuprofen and Katie seemed to rally, played outside, and ate her supper of macaroni and cheese with no problems. Katie took her bath and went upstairs to bed for stories at her regular time, and went to sleep without any fuss. Around midnight, I heard a commotion upstairs, and when I went into her bedroom to investigate, I found that Katie was vomiting just as I arrived. We changed the sheets and washed her up, and she went back to sleep. She was still warm, but not enough to cause alarm. Both of the girls had been sick before, and we weren't all that worried. Parents with small children see it frequently, and get used to it. Katie woke up Saturday morning, still sick, but not seriously ill. Cheryl and I didn't know how sick she really was.

On Saturdays, our schedule was more relaxed than during the week. Katie felt too sick to eat her breakfast. She just lounged on the couch, watched a few of her favorite cartoon TV shows, and rested. Cheryl was watching her temperature closely and found that it was higher this morning. She gave her more ibuprofen, and when the temperature stayed up, reaching 104 degrees, Cheryl called the pediatrician's office for counsel. They told us that the duration of the fever, though high in temperature, was not enough to warrant an office visit. They concluded she probably had a viral infection that would pass in twenty-four hours or so. Again, this was nothing out of the ordinary.

I decided to go to work for a few hours and Cheryl agreed to call me if anything changed. Katie went to lie down in the big bed in our bedroom and fell asleep around noon. This in itself was a red flag, as she hadn't gone to sleep in the middle of the day since she was two years old. Katie had boundless energy and refused to nap for fear that she would miss some adventure. This had caused problems at her daycare, as she was the only child who refused to lie down at nap time. She wanted to go for a walk or play basketball—anything except rest. At home, when her sister was napping, we had to pay special attention to Katie to keep her occupied and quiet so Molly could sleep.

I returned home around three thirty in the afternoon and found Katie still sleeping and still feverish. At four she woke up and moved from the big bed to the couch in the living room. Her temperature was still up and it was time for more medicine. Even with another dose, her fever did not come down as it should.

Katie did not want to eat supper, but she was drinking fluids and keeping them down without vomiting. She told us she wasn't hungry, but she did want to take a bath. Bath time was fun for the girls, and when Katie was younger, she would splash and kick so much that we would get soaking wet, too. But we made it fun and just found a dry shirt when it was over.

Today was my mother's birthday and Cheryl had made a cake for her. After we had eaten supper, we agreed that I would give the girls their baths and Cheryl would run over to my mother's house with the cake and a birthday card. She had not been able to go in the afternoon because Katie had been sleeping.

I gave Molly her bath first, and then I helped Katie with hers. She seemed to enjoy it and play and have as much fun as when she wasn't sick, but when the time came to get out and dry off, Katie refused to get out of the tub. She told me that she liked her bath, and she liked her house, and she did not want to get out of the tub ever again. The water was cooling off and I thought she should get out and get ready for bed. I played along, thinking she liked it because she was so hot. Eventually I decided it was time to get her out, and I had to reach in and pick her up to do it. I had never had to do this before; it was always possible to coax her out and into a towel, by making a game out of it. Not this night.

We had had some trouble getting Katie, always energetic, to go sleep for more than a year, and we found that a solid routine made it easier. The schedule consisted of suppertime around five, with a bath immediately following, and pajamas on by six. That way Katie and Molly could visit with Cheryl, who typically arrived home from work around six during the week. Sometimes they watched TV for a bit, and would start up to bed for stories at six thirty and lights out at seven.

One night during the summer, after all the bedtime work was done and I had finished the last story with Katie, I turned off the light in her bedroom and lay back down in her bed to comfort her until she fell asleep. This was a concession we had made, against the advice of the psychology pantheon, to prevent her from screaming at bedtime. Katie did not want to be separated from us and bedtime was no different. She was a strong-willed child and insisted that one of us stay with her, patting her back or humming a good-night lullaby until she fell asleep. If we did not stay, she would scream and cry and wake up her sister, and it would go on for an hour or more. But if one of us lay down for a few minutes with her, she would fall right asleep.

On that ordinary night in the summer, Katie, without prompting, turned to me and said, "I love my room, Dad. I love my house. And I love you." The thought went through my mind that I hoped I could sustain her room and her house for her. Being self-employed in a physically demanding field, I was always worried about getting hurt and not being able to work and make enough money for the mortgage payment. It was a comfort to me to know she was happy in her surroundings. In the months to follow, that thought would mean more than I understood at the time.

That September Saturday, after I picked Katie up out of the tub and got her dressed, she just sat on the couch, obviously not feeling well. She soon developed a barking cough and complained of a pain in her stomach. She said that she just wanted to go to bed, to go up to her room, the place she loved and where she felt so comfortable.

I took her upstairs while Cheryl, who had just arrived back home, called the doctor's office. As Katie sat on the edge of her bed getting ready for a bedtime story, I noticed that she was breathing especially hard. She complained again of a sharp pain in her stomach. Every now and then she would emit a barklike cough and her nostrils would flare.

7

Cheryl, still on the phone with the doctor's office trying to figure out what to do, came upstairs to Katie's room. When I saw Katie's nostrils flare with each breath, I immediately decided to take her to the hospital in Concord, which was thirty-five minutes away. Salisbury is a rural town about twenty-five miles northwest of Concord, New Hampshire, with a population of fourteen hundred residents. The hospital in Concord serves our town and many other surrounding towns. Katie left the room and the house that she loved so much at seven thirty on September 22, my mother's birthday.

CHAPTER 2

Katie

Katie was born on Halloween, a healthy child of seven pounds, seven ounces. Cheryl had a three-month maternity leave, which was a big help for us getting used to our first baby. When Cheryl went back to work, I stayed home for the rest of the winter with Katie. Staying home all day was a big change for me. It kept me cooped up in the house all winter and demanded a mostly sedentary workday. Still, I was happy to be able to spend so much time with my little girl and we became close.

Katie grew fast and became big for her age, in the ninety-ninth percentile for head circumference, length, and weight. Because she was so big, she started to walk later than the typical toddler, at twenty months. For the first year and a half Katie was content to sit or lie quietly, without struggling to move, roll over, learn to walk, or even stand up. This late start in her physical development belied the energy that she would later exhibit.

Her verbal development was delayed as well, though she made plenty of noise and was able to communicate effectively with her parents and caregivers. Katie's pediatrician suggested that she receive some speech therapy to investigate if there were further problems in that area, so we signed her up for a program through the hospital. In Katie's case, the explosion of language that her pediatrician told us would occur didn't happen until she was more than four years old. At age four, she was eligible to be enrolled in the preschool speech therapy program, and she attended school two days per week for two and a half hours in the morning.

The teachers at this preschool had their hands full with their new student. Katie was unruly and resisted settling down into the structure of the classroom. She was highly social and virtually ignored the teachers if there was something she decided she was going to do. In an attempt to impress upon her the consequences of acting up, the teachers would threaten to bring her to the principal's office. Katie jumped at the chance, grabbing the hand of the teacher and leading her out the door and down the hall to the office. She missed the whole point of the exercise and was not the least bit afraid to enjoy the next adventure of meeting the principal.

She became the informal classroom greeter, welcoming the other students as they arrived, helping them to take off their coats and get ready for class. In group activities she sat at the head of the table, ready to lead her classmates in whatever task was assigned to them. When the halls were empty, the preschool students would ride a large purple tricycle up and down the hallway while the teachers studied their motor skills. Katie loved the tricycle and mastered it right away. She would pedal fast, quickly outpacing the teachers, and ride all the way down to the other end of the building, cackling and giggling, with the teachers chasing her, trying to get her to turn around and come back to the preschool end of the building. Nothing worked. She was her own person.

Katie was an emotional child. She was closely attached to us and especially so to me. She became anxious any time she felt that she would be separated from us. Cheryl commuted for an hour to her full-time job and an hour home every day, so she was out the door early. I was a self-employed building contractor and could set my own work hours, so I was the one who took Katie and Molly to and from the daycare and school.

On many mornings, after I succeeded in getting Katie dressed and focused my attention on Molly, I would turn around to find Katie totally naked and running around the house, giggling and dancing. I had both hands full with her.

In the more formal daycare settings and preschool, Katie caused an absolute scene when I dropped her off, screaming and holding my leg.

It became a little game to get her interested in her surroundings and start her playing with her schoolmates. Dropping her off became an event that took half an hour most days. Her teachers were used to this behavior and were pretty good sports at getting her focused, tolerating her outbursts and the "drop down," where she would fall to the floor and scream. She was quite social once we were out of sight, but clearly she was not the average child.

Katie's speech was still not developing at a pace with which everyone was comfortable, so her teachers started looking at other possibilities for the cause of the delay. That summer, I made an appointment with a specialty clinic in Manchester to explore the causes, including the possibility of an autism spectrum disorder.

Katie's first visit to the clinic was a hoot; she went from office to office introducing herself to staff members. "Hi, I'm Katie," she said. "What's your name?" During one of the diagnostic testing procedures, one of the doctors asked her to name different pictures in a book, with progressively harder concepts. As it became harder for her, Katie became frustrated, and suddenly pushed the book back across the table at him. "I'm done," she said. When he tried to coax her into continuing the exercise, she slammed the book shut, slid it across the table to him, and said, quite firmly, "I'm done!" We both chuckled, and the doctor remarked that he had never before been dismissed by a four-year-old.

Though no firm diagnosis could be made from the clinic visits, several things could be ruled out, including mental retardation and autism. After the last visit I had a few extra minutes, so I took her around the corner to the same Irish pub that I used to frequent when I was in college. The same bartender was still there, remembered my name, and shouted, "Johnny! Where you been, lad?" It had been at least ten years since I had set foot inside that pub.

Without asking, he drew a pint of Guinness and put it on the counter in front of me. I asked him if Katie could sit at the bar with me. Since it was two thirty in the afternoon on a weekday and there was nobody there, he said it was okay. She sat right up on a bar stool, drinking a chocolate milk and eating chicken nuggets, chatting with the bartender, fully enjoying this new adventure. She was with her dad, and was at home anyplace as long as she was with me.

Katie returned to preschool when the new school year began in late August. Classes three days a week instead of two, and now in the afternoon, proved to be a big load for a four-year-old. When I picked her up on school days, she would fall asleep in the truck before we left the parking lot. On these days she would often go to bed early, on her own, something she had never done. I thought she was getting physically run down from all her activities, and I worried about it. We had taken her to the experts and nothing serious was found, so we accepted that it was part of her growing up and was normal.

CHAPTER 3

Going to the Hospital

At the time I decided to take Katie to the hospital, we didn't understand what was wrong with our little girl. Cheryl and I had both assumed she had croup, would get some antibiotics, and come home that night. I went in my work clothes, throwing on a clean t-shirt on the way out the door, and told Cheryl that I would call her as soon as I found out what was happening. Cheryl dressed Katie in her jacket and slippers, followed us out to the car, and said to Katie, "I love you, Katie." There was a tone in her voice that night that is hard to describe. I had never heard it in eight years of marriage.

That was the moment we both realized that this could be a serious illness, but it still seemed only a possibility. Neither of us really believed it. The worry of serious illness is always in the back of a parent's mind when fever strikes their babies, but in the era of modern medicine, we never believe the unthinkable will happen. We had good health insurance, the hospital we were going to was a good one, and in New England, a great hospital is not much more than an hour away.

When we arrived at the hospital, I opened the back door of the car, reached inside to pick her up, and started to carry her. After I had gone about three steps, Katie declared that she wanted to walk. I told her it was okay, that I would carry her. "No, Daddy," she said, "I can walk." So, Katie, as sick as she was, walked with me into the emergency department at Concord Hospital, holding my hand.

When we arrived inside at eight fifteen on a Saturday night with a nearly full moon, we found the ED crowded and busy. Concord is a city of forty thousand residents, and the hospital serves the surrounding communities for about twenty-five miles in all directions. It's a high-volume emergency department and treats everything from sore throats and auto accidents to the homeless population and geriatric patients. That night almost all the chairs were full of waiting patients. Many of them appeared to be suffering from emotional problems, as some of them were literally howling at the moon, talking to themselves, or moaning and uttering strange noises.

The protocol requires that a little green form be filled out with the patient's information and a description of the problem. A nurse behind a window takes the form and assigns a number to the patient. Then one sits in the waiting room and waits to be called, not unlike the deli at the supermarket. That night a sharp triage nurse was working at the desk. When she saw a little girl who looked very sick, she came right out and said, "Come with me." Katie had a pallor to her face that indicated she was not getting enough oxygen, and though I didn't notice it, the nurse did.

As we went through the door into the triage area, I heard the nurse talking into a portable phone, and the words I heard gave me chills. "I need respiratory to triage, *stat*. I need a physician to triage, *stat*, I need radiology to triage, *stat*." My mother was a registered nurse for forty years. When she got mad and wanted her children to do something quickly, her request was followed by the exclamation, "*Stat!*" The word, the abbreviated form of the Latin *statim*, means something that must be done without delay. The nurse knew that Katie needed immediate attention. I knew what it meant but still did not believe that my little girl was that sick. After all, she had just walked across the parking lot with me.

The nurse put an oxygen mask on Katie while another one recorded the history of her sickness as I related it. Fever for just over twenty-four hours, high fever of 104 for twelve hours, ibuprofen and acetaminophen given for twenty-four hours, vomiting one time eighteen hours earlier, no recent vomiting, fluids staying down, sleeping for three hours during the day, barklike cough for one hour, stomach cramps for one hour, nostrils flaring for one hour, walking into the ED. That was it. With no previous history, Katie was a healthy kid. But she wasn't healthy right now.

The nurse attached a small probe to one of Katie's fingers, the kind with a little spring in it, like a clothespin, to hold it in place. The probe is attached to a pulse oximeter, which records the oxygen levels in the hemoglobin, the protein in the blood that carries oxygen. This tells the caregiver whether or not the lungs are functioning properly at their job of getting oxygen into the blood, usually at least 95 percent. The pulse oximeter revealed that Katie's oxygen saturation was below normal, at 86 percent. The oxygen mask brought it back up into the high nineties, and she looked and felt much better.

Katie was sitting up in the hospital bed, and I was at her bedside holding her hand now and then. Katie was an independent child and did not always feel the need to hold hands. She was having trouble keeping the oxygen mask on, so I helped her hold it in place while we waited for the doctor. Unbeknownst to me, the doctor was already working on her case, arranging the next step. While we waited, Katie kept removing the oxygen mask, saying, "I'm done." One of the nurses was watching and came over with a teddy bear. Then the nurse replaced the mask with a nostril tube and Katie seemed to like it better. It was not as claustrophobic as the mask, and she could look around; she didn't want to miss anything.

As the nurses hovered around Katie's bed, more and more people entered and exited the room. Nasal swabs were taken and sent off to the lab. A portable X-ray machine was produced and chest X-rays were taken of her lungs. The X-rays, called films in the medical profession, showed an opaque white area of approximately 50 percent of her right lung, but her left lung was clear. Once the X-rays were taken, they moved us from the first triage area to an area closer to the doors leading to the ambulance docks. I thought this was odd, as sick patients are usually moved in the other direction, toward the hospital rooms, when being considered for admission. I didn't know at the time that this meant that, if possible, they would not keep such a sick child at a small general hospital like Concord.

Once we moved out of triage and into the rear area of the ambulance dock, the nurses flitted in and out of Katie's curtained-off room. None of them knew, or would say if they did know, exactly what was going on with Katie. They offered the usual platitudes of "She looks so much better," or "Can I get you anything while we wait for the doctor?" I sensed that something was amiss.

After a few minutes, the doctor, Geoff, appeared and introduced himself to me, carrying the chest films in a big yellow envelope. He told me that Katie was very sick and that Concord Hospital did not have the resources to deal with what she had. He told me that there were three hospitals in New England that could offer the level of care that Katie needed. One in Lebanon, New Hampshire, one in Portland, Maine, and one in Boston, Massachusetts. I was stunned and asked, "Doctor, how sick is she?"

"Katie is the sickest patient in New Hampshire tonight, and when she gets to where she is going, she will be the sickest patient in the United States."

I couldn't believe what I was hearing, I thought that I must be missing some big part of the picture. I asked him what was wrong, and he told me that Katie had a dangerously aggressive type of bacterial pneumonia, and she needed to go to a bigger hospital that could help her better than they could there. Her sickness was not the croup.

He outlined the options for transfer and asked if I had any preferences. I replied that my sister's husband had been recently diagnosed with leukemia and was currently a patient at the hospital in Lebanon, New Hampshire. Since my sister was traveling up to Lebanon every day, I thought it was logical that we bring Katie to that hospital, so that we could share rides and have some family present to help support each other. It was also the closest of the three options. I didn't know at the time that this was the same doctor who had diagnosed my brother-in-law just two weeks before, and transferred him with only hours to live. By correctly diagnosing him and taking quick action, he had already saved the life of one our family members. Tonight, he was trying to do it again.

He called the hospital in Lebanon and discovered that they were full. Since Portland is two and half hours away, Boston, at one and a half hours away, was my next choice. Cheryl's sister, Debbie, is a medical doctor, and lived in Boston then, so we would have some family support there if we needed it. Boston had a bed open and the doctor told me that the helicopter was already in the air and would be landing in about twenty minutes to take us to the bigger hospital. He also told me that I needed to go with Katie in the helicopter and to make my arrangements, which my doctor friend tells me is not usually the case when transferring adults. He placed the chest films on Katie's bed, said, "Don't lose these," and shook my hand.

A helicopter. Already in the air. This *was* serious. It was now ten o'clock, and I had to move fast. I called Chris, my younger brother, who lived a few miles away from us in Salisbury, to get him headed my way, to take the car home to Cheryl. Then I called Cheryl and told her what we were doing. She was at home with Molly, who was asleep, and didn't want to drive my truck to Boston and meet us. Then I called my mother, Ruthann. My mother and father lived in an in-law apartment attached to my brother's house. My brother, my sister Heidi, and I were all close to my mother, and in times of family crisis she often served as the call center and dispatch. We called her and told her what was happening, and she relayed information as it was needed. Over the next three weeks she would prove to be invaluable in this role.

My brother and his wife arrived in record time and watched as the flight nurse wheeled the gurney across the parking lot to the helipad. They opened the back door of the helicopter and slid Katie in on the gurney, just like in a regular ambulance. There was a bench on each side of the gurney inside the cabin. I tossed him the car keys, climbed aboard the helicopter, strapped myself in, and donned a helmet with a set of headphones so I could communicate with the flight nurses and the pilot, still in stunned disbelief that this was happening. At no point in the next three weeks would I feel as though I fully understood what was happening to Katie or to our family. We were at the mercy of the system. In an instant, I had become a stranger in a strange land.

I had a few minutes to rest and think, contemplating our new adventure as the chopper made its way south. I had no idea what was coming, what it all meant, where it would end. I sent a text message to my friend in North Carolina, a retired college professor and administrator, who always laughed at the crazy things that happened to me. It felt like I was bobbing along a fast-moving river with no paddle or rudder. Katie was lying on the gurney next to me, holding my hand occasionally, but wasn't talking much. She was tired and was resting, not aware of what was going on around her. If she had been healthy, a helicopter ride would have been the highlight of her day. She would have wanted a parachute so she could jump out and squeal all the way to the ground.

CHAPTER 4

Boston Emergency Department

As the helicopter descended to the well-lit rooftop, I could see a security guard and several people in white lab coats standing outside a double-wide glass door. The people at the glass door ran over to the helipad as the flight nurse moved quickly to open the doors and unstrap the gurney. I unbuckled my seat belt, opened my door, and jumped out onto the roof into a nearly blinding rotor wash, ducking my head in fear of the still-moving rotors. The engine noise was deafening. As soon as Katie's stretcher was free, the lab coat people and the flight nurse grabbed it and started power walking toward the open doors. They were speaking in medical terms to each other, a language I did not understand, though some English words made their way into the discourse. No one said a word to me and I was afraid they would leave me behind if I didn't keep up with them. The group was moving fast, almost running, talking as fast as they were moving. I felt like I was running to catch up, in more ways than one.

We entered a labyrinth of hallways, elevators, and glass-covered skybridges that wound down into the belly of the hospital. As we traveled through the buildings, at every door a respectful and attentive security guard or two held it open for the entourage. Every elevator door was open on the right floor, with another guard holding it for the people moving so fast with a sick little girl. I was completely lost. At last, the elevator door opened, and we stepped from one world into another. We had arrived on the first floor of the hospital in the emergency department at eleven thirty on a Saturday night.

They wheeled Katie into the biggest triage room I had ever seen. It had curtains that could be slid around on tracks in the ceiling, so the room could be partitioned off to handle multiple trauma cases at once. On this night, however, all of the curtains were pulled back against the walls, allowing use of the entire room. I had never before seen so many people in one room in a hospital. Every person wore a yellow gown with a matching mask on their face. With so many people from so many different disciplines in such close quarters, the opportunity for chaos should have been ripe. But there was no chaos; here there was a disciplined, well-organized operation, fully prepared to handle our medical emergency. Each person knew exactly what to do and knew the exact function of every other person in the room. There was total silence. They were all looking at us.

Katie was still conscious, though breathing heavily. I was holding her hand and talking to her. I told her that she would be okay, that all these people were here to help her. I asked her if she was scared and she shook her head, and firmly said, "No." Then she patted my hand and said, "You'll be okay, Daddy." Here in the ED was a sick little girl telling her dad *he* would be okay. It appeared to me that Katie was losing consciousness, that she was fading in and out and getting sicker, though by now her oxygen saturation was up to 97 percent.

As the doctors began their work, one of them started interviewing me to get the background on Katie. I stepped away from Katie's bedside, assuring her that everything would be all right. As the medications started to take effect, she drifted off to sleep. Afraid that it might be the last that I saw of Katie as I knew her, I didn't want to leave, but I had to get out of the way.

The lead doctor in the ED wanted to know everything I could tell her, and I did my best to relate the story of Katie's brief sickness. She asked me if we had chickens, and was there any chance that Katie had been exposed to their droppings. Puzzled, I answered no, and asked her why. She told me that sometimes bird droppings contain bacteria that could cause pneumonia symptoms similar to Katie's. I asked her what she thought it was, and she told me that they didn't know for sure, except that they thought it was an aggressive type of bacterial pneumonia.

It was now after eleven thirty and I was starting to get tired. When I had finished briefing the doctor, a woman put her hand on my shoulder and introduced herself. She was a social worker and had come to the ED to offer her assistance to me as the father and walking wounded. She brought a chair for me and suggested that I sit down. Of course, I could not sit down, as upset as I was, but I appreciated the thought and her offer. She was a true professional, concerned for Katie and for me, too, and offered to get me anything I needed. At this point, what I needed was a long drink of water, which she found for me in warm half-pint bottles. It would do.

As I stood in the back of the emergency room I could see and hear the buzz of activity around Katie. There was no shouting, only quiet, rapid talking. One person stood at a computer on a mobile cart about six feet away from the foot of Katie's bed, and entered everything that was being done into the chart. She was busy. I watched as one person cut Katie's brand-new t-shirt off with a pair of scissors. Katie loved those new shirts; she wanted to wear them all the time. They were boy's size six, the only ones we could find that fit her well. If Cheryl knew that the hospital staff had cut that shirt up, she would have had a fit. It was a fitting irony, because Katie would sometimes cut her own shirts, or her hair, or Molly's hair, or her pants, or the drapes, or the couch cover, with her children's scissors, just for fun, or to practice cutting, as she would say. Katie would have approved.

I heard a voice over the hospital loudspeaker say, "Anesthesia to ED, *stat*, Respiratory to ED, *stat*," and minutes later several men in lab coats with stethoscopes around their necks came running down the hallway and into the room. As I conversed with the social worker about what was happening, I started counting the number of people in the room. There were fifty-six people already there, and every few minutes one or two more would arrive. It soon became so crowded that there was no room for me and the social worker, so we stepped out into the hallway. I could no longer see Katie. She was hidden behind a wall of yellow gowns and white lab coats, every one of them trying to get a handle on her sickness and do what they could to save her life.

I had now been awake for twenty hours. I sat down in the chair.

CHAPTER 5

Seven South

The ED staff determined that Katie was in acute respiratory distress. There was a type of pneumonia in her lungs preventing the proper exchange of oxygen and blood gases, and the affected area was growing. Some type of bacteria had settled into her lungs and was blocking her body's absorption of oxygen.

Though Katie was very sick, the doctors felt she was stable enough to be moved to the Pediatric Intensive Care Unit, or PICU, located in the south wing of the seventh floor of the hospital. There the PICU staff would be able to do extensive testing and examination and could dig in for the long run if that became necessary.

The ED staff had started IV lines of medication, but Katie was still breathing on her own, and her oxygen saturation rate was stable. They decided to intubate her there in the ED, however, in case she suddenly got worse. The doctor would insert a tube into Katie's mouth that would allow easier and faster access to the lungs for the breathing and suction machines, should they be required. Katie would not be able to talk, but she was now heavily medicated and would feel no pain. I thought that the doctor was almost asking for my permission without actually posing the question, and I assured her that I wanted her to do whatever she felt was needed to help my daughter. The intubation tube was inserted and more medications were ordered and plugged into Katie's IVs while we talked outside the room.

At last, the sea of yellow gowns and white lab coats parted and Katie was wheeled out of the ED and toward the elevators for the short ride to the seventh floor. A large group of doctors and nurses escorted Katie's hospital bed, attending to her during the transit. There were anesthesia doctors, IV nurses, the recording nurse, and a host of other medical professionals within inches of her bed during the transit. Not a word was spoken that did not involve the care of Katie during the transition to the PICU. I was invited to go along and the social worker came with us. She was assigned to the ED and her shift ended at midnight, a few minutes away. She could have wished me well and said goodbye as I left for the seventh floor, but instead, she volunteered to come with us, and stayed by my side as we headed out and up.

Moving a critically ill patient with IVs from one floor to another in a hospital is a big job. It requires close attention to the rolling IV stands and extra care to avoid obstacles in the hallways that might impede progress, or worse, tangle a line and hurt the patient. The members of the transport staff were professionals and made it look easy. There was no shouting, only determined and serious attention to the job at hand. Her room was located near the nurse's station on Seven South, and Katie was wheeled into a smaller space than the ED offered, but with no shortage of technology.

Throughout the walk, the social worker kept explaining to me where we were, who was whom, and where we were going. I felt as though she should be holding an oil lantern and dressed in a hooded monk's robe, and that the others present could not see us, but that we could see them. She was my guide and I the observer, and I was being given a privileged tour of something mortals were not allowed to witness this side of Hades. She was cool, an experienced medical professional, but not distant, displaying a demeanor that can only come from someone who has seen terrible things happen to children many, many times.

Day 2. 12:02 a.m., Sunday, September 23: The PICU

The first person I met on Seven South was the nurse who ran the chart computer. Her job was to oversee the recording of the data on Katie as it was ordered by the doctors and administered by the nurses. She was bubbly and energetic, while staying focused on her role.

Her post was at a computer at the foot of Katie's bed, and now I began to understand what that person in the ED was doing. As medications were ordered, she entered them into the electronic chart: time, dosage, and name of the doctor who ordered it. As the meds were hooked up and plugged in, first into the infusion pump and then into Katie's veins, the nurse entered that the order had been completed. This created an accurate record of what went on and made it immediately available electronically throughout the entire hospital.

A picture began to emerge of what was wrong with Katie. She had a lung infection, a type of pneumonia, but not the regular kind. This pneumonia was virulent and moving quickly. It was now known that she tested positive for methicillin-resistant *Staphylococcus aureus*. MRSA is a contagious, dangerous, fast-moving, and life-threatening bacteria. It was in the lungs of my little girl, and was spreading rapidly.

On the skin and in the blood, there is treatment to combat MRSA. In the lung, however, it is nearly impossible to treat. Doctors call it necrotizing pneumonia, meaning that the bacteria are actually killing the cells in the lung, causing permanent damage. I didn't know much about medicine or medical terminology at the time, but the expressions on the faces of the doctors and nurses told me her condition was very serious.

One of the doctors came out of the fray to talk to me about Katie, and introduced herself as one of the fellows. She told me that Katie was very sick with bacterial pneumonia and the doctors were treating her with antibiotics. I had to learn the nomenclature and hierarchy of doctors in a teaching hospital. The terms I knew as a layman had different meanings in an academic hospital setting, terms like resident, fellow, and attending.

The differences among resident, fellow, and attending physicians can be described something like this. A resident is a doctor who has graduated from four years of medical school, after graduating from four years of college, and has earned the title of medical doctor. One then becomes a resident in a specialty area, such as pediatrics, which requires three years of study, or surgery, which requires five years of study, generally, to be able to sit for the various certification exams. A fellow is one who chooses a subspecialty course of study after residency, generally consisting of up to three years of additional training in that specialty. An attending physician is one who has completed all the training and subspecialty training, and is now in independent practice. It takes a lot of education to become a medical doctor. I felt out of place in the company of these highly educated people, but they explained things in a compassionate way so that I could understand them.

12:15 a.m., Sunday, September 23:
First Code

Without warning, at twelve fifteen, now Sunday morning, Katie's monitors sprang to life with alarms. A strobe light outside the room began flashing and people started running toward where we were standing outside of Katie's room. The fellow excused herself and jumped into the fracas at the bedside.

A tall doctor was ordering medications in a precise and measured way to those around Katie's bed. The room, and then the hallway, began to fill up with doctors and nurses. I kept stepping back farther and farther away from Katie's room, allowing the staff to get in close and do their jobs. My social worker and guide remained calm, and when I asked her what was happening, explained that Katie's vital signs had dropped a little lower than what was considered safe. Katie was receiving medications to help her body regain adequate levels of function. What the social worker did not tell me, either because she did not know or because she did not want me to hear it from anyone other than a doctor, was that Katie's heart had almost stopped, and a rescue dose of epinephrine had been administered to bring her back. I did not learn about this until much later in the evening, and when I learned it, I still did not know what it meant. I thought epinephrine was for bee stings, an accurate indication of my ignorance about medical procedures.

I had never been in an intensive care unit as an observer before that night. I had undergone surgery several times, in a regular room each time. Through the haze of medication, a patient can't really see what is happening around him. I thought that what was going on with Katie was standard protocol in a big hospital. I thought at first that the large group assembled in the ED had been a false alarm, that Katie was not as sick as we might have thought. She was sick, to be sure, but in the ED just downstairs half an hour ago, she was conscious and still able to communicate. It began to dawn on me that Katie was indeed in a dire situation, and her condition did require all those people around her. She had arrived in the PICU not a moment too soon.

I had picked up a few medical phrases from my mother over the years, phrases that I had forgotten about until that night. "Frank blood," meaning fresh blood, was one of them, and the nurse in charge of operating the suction machine attached to Katie repeated the phrase several times, followed by the amount "one hundred CCs," and more. I watched the suction cup at the head of Katie's bed and I was horrified when at last I realized that the liquid pouring into that cup was fluid mixed with blood, and it was coming from my little girl's lungs. When asked by the doctor in charge, the nurse continued repeating "frank blood," and then started to repeat "copious amounts," another phrase I had learned from my mother. Copious amounts of frank blood meant that Katie was bleeding to death through her lungs.

The suction cup was filling up. Where was it all coming from, I wondered? At only fifty-two pounds, this little girl did not have a lot of blood in her body. I became sick to my stomach. It was at that point

I realized that not only was Katie as sick as the first doctor at Concord Hospital had told me, but in fact she might die, and soon.

As Katie's condition deteriorated and more people crowded around, I moved farther away from the door to Katie's room. At one point I was standing directly behind the attending physician, who was closely monitoring everything as it happened, when her portable hospital phone rang. She answered it and calmly said, "May I call you back? I am in the middle of a code." I had heard my mother talk about codes and I didn't know what one looked like, but my daughter was now the cause of a code. I did not know what was going on. The attending physician would tell me later that night, "She tried to die on us in there."

Standing outside of the room with my social worker and guide, I started counting heads again. There were twenty-four people in the room, with another twenty-eight people standing in the hallway. Fifty-two highly trained and compassionate souls and not a peep from any of them. It was so quiet that the alarms and the few people talking in Katie's room could be clearly heard from where I was, twenty feet away, through the open doors and outside the room. None of them looked at me or even acknowledged that I was there. They were intently focused on the patient, watching, waiting, standing by to assist in whatever capacity was needed. The look on their faces spoke for them: everyone wore a visage of grave concern that can only be seen in a pediatric intensive care unit during a code.

To a parent in a hospital ward with an acutely ill child, time seems to stand still. I felt like I had entered a zone that was not bound by any schedules or deadlines, that time as one of our standard laws had been suspended. I would occasionally glance at the clock on the wall or my cell phone, but I had no sensation of time. It was simply a different number or location of the hands on the clock face, as though time had been transformed into nothing more than an irrelevant construct. And I was tired.

After a period of this new time standard, things began to calm down in Katie's room. Her vital signs returned to a more normal range and she stabilized. Then the fellow came out to tell me that Katie was now better, that she was receiving the proper medications and her condition looked positive. It was now approaching one in the morning and my social worker asked me if I was going to be okay. I told her yes, that she should go home, and she agreed to go, but only if I felt strong enough to be by myself. At no point during the evening, or in my entire adult life, for that matter, had I ever not felt strong enough to be by myself. Most of the time I prefer to be alone anyway. Still, it was reassuring to have an insider with me to identify the different phases of Katie's early hospitalization.

Most social workers that I knew from academia tended to be the touchy-feely type, those who, when listening to someone speak, cock their heads to one side, look deep into their eyes, nod their heads a lot, and reply with "uh-hum," or "I see." This social worker was not like that, and her behavior could only have been acquired from gritty, real-world experience. The presence of this social worker and her successor was a tremendous gift from the hospital. It proved to be the first of many that we would receive.

I stepped outside the immediate area into a back hallway to call Cheryl and tell her that Katie had coded, but was back from the brink. I told her to get some sleep, but instead of coming to Boston in the morning, I wanted her to take Molly to our pediatrician's office and get her tested. I needed to know if Molly's little cold was the same germ that was wreaking such havoc on Katie, and if so, I wanted to catch it before it got this bad. Cheryl agreed and I told her I would call if anything changed.

I returned to the area outside Katie's room. Things were still quiet. There was a bench in the back of her hospital room with a few blankets and pillows, and the nurses told me to lie down and get some rest. They promised to be quiet. I had been awake for twenty-one hours and I was getting tired.

2:05 a.m., Sunday, September 23:
Second Code and Pneumothorax

I lay down on the bench for about an hour. I couldn't sleep. It was busy and bright in the room and there was a lot of background noise. Nurses were in and out every few minutes and Katie's room remained a center of activity. Suddenly the monitor alarms started again. The lights were turned way up and a flood of people entered the room. Doctors and nurses crowded around Katie's bed as before, with the same drill taking place. I had no idea what was going on. I got up from the bench and worked my way outside into the hallway. I was in the way, and worried that I was impeding the work of the staff.

The fellow told me that Katie had developed a tension pneumo-thorax, a condition caused by a leak in the lung, sometimes called a collapsed lung. Air enters the pleural or chest cavity with each inhaled breath, but can't escape with the exhaled breath. It creates tension and the difference in air pressure soon causes the lung to be compressed, preventing proper gas exchange of oxygen and carbon dioxide.

The medical team decided to insert a chest tube on her left side to relieve the pressure building up inside her chest cavity. A chest tube is literally a tube inserted between the ribs into the pleural cavity, and it allows any buildup of air or fluid to be drained away from the lung. There is a one-way valve used on the tube that prevents air from re-entering the chest cavity. It's called a Heimlich valve, named for its inventor, Dr. Henry Heimlich, whom most of us know from his other contribution to medicine, the Heimlich maneuver.

The fellow inserted the chest tube into Katie's left fourth intercostal space, resulting in a gush of air and a small amount of blood. More bedside attention went on for about an hour, and then Katie stabilized, just like before.

The tall doctor now took the time to speak to me. He asked me how I was doing and I told him that I was a little tired, but that otherwise I was fine. I asked him what was going on with Katie. He gave me a precise rundown on the procedures that the team was conducting on her. He described the care being given to her neurological and other states, and the medications used to address each of the needs. He then asked me if I had been told what all of this treatment meant. I told him that I really did not understand what was happening.

He said that many parents feel that way and some are difficult to communicate with about medical terms. He said he thought that I was pretty sharp, but that I had simply not been informed. I told him that many procedures had been explained to me in rather scientific and medical terms, but it looked to me like Katie was dying. He said that in fact Katie had come close on two occasions, but that medications were being given to prevent that from happening. I asked him about the copious amounts of blood that were still pouring into the cup from the suction machine. He said that the blood and serous fluid being drained from Katie's lungs was serious but manageable, and that Katie's lab reports and blood chemistry concerning oxygen levels and antibiotics indicated progress. He told me to lie down and try to get some sleep.

The tall doctor was in charge for the night and his keen intellect and calm behavior during the codes showed a man who was in control of a nearly uncontrollable situation. He never got rattled, never shouted, and when things had stabilized, sought me out on his own to explain it to me as best he could. He displayed a genuine concern for Katie and for me. The other doctors told me later that he was the one who "captured" Katie that night. To capture a patient means to keep them from dying.

5:20 a.m., Sunday, September 23:
Third Code

I lay down on the bench again and almost on cue, Katie coded once more. It was now after five on Sunday morning. I got up and went outside the room, and the fellow came out to talk to me. She asked me where the child's mother was and told me that I should call her and instruct her to come to the hospital as soon as possible. She said to me, "I do not know where this is going," referring to Katie's deteriorating condition, a phrase she repeated several times. I couldn't believe what I was hearing. It made me realize that Katie's condition was not only as bad as I thought and had been told, but was getting worse, and we might lose her. I had to move fast. I had to call Cheryl and tell her what was happening, that Katie was fading, tell her what the doctor had told me, and get her heading to Boston as soon as she could.

I stepped out through the double doors and into the hallway that connects the PICU to the elevator area and called Cheryl again. I told her that it was clear that Katie was much sicker than we thought, that Katie might die, and soon, and that she should be here with us if that happened. It came as a shock, in the short five hours since we arrived in Boston, and was difficult for both of us to comprehend. I don't remember the exact words we exchanged, but I told her that they were losing Katie, that she was dying, and that she should get Molly up and head for Boston. I told her to call me when she was on the road and I would find somebody to give her directions when she got close. I had arrived by helicopter and had no idea how to get to the hospital in a car. She understood, and though she was as upset as I was, she headed for Boston as soon as we hung up.

I then called my mother and told her that Katie was fading. I knew it would upset her, but I knew she should be aware that we could lose Katie that night.

It was time to bring in the family support network and I started with the ones who were closest geographically. I called Cheryl's parents, Jim and Ann, and asked them to come to Boston to help us with Molly and to see Katie in case things went bad. I also called Cheryl's sister, Debbie. She is a medical doctor and lived in South Boston at the time, about two miles away from the hospital. I was starting to get worn out, with no sleep for almost twenty-four hours and a beautiful daughter who was dying before my eyes. I spoke to Debbie's fiancé, Tim, first. He was taken totally by surprise, being awakened in the early morning and having no knowledge that Katie was sick or that we were in Boston. But he could tell I wasn't kidding, that things were bad.

Debbie and Tim arrived first, at about six, and were the first to offer support. The look on their faces gave them away. The are both medical professionals, and what they saw made them sick with worry. I was in tough shape by this time and Tim did his best to comfort his macho future brother-in-law.

Debbie looked at Tim, then they both looked at me, and she said, "What is happening here? Did you see that board?" I didn't know what board she was talking about, until one of the nurses pulled it out from underneath Katie as she laid in her hospital bed. It was a piece of white plastic that looked sort of like the backboard that one uses in rescue operations in the field, but smaller. I had lifted a few people onto back-boards over the years, and I had done cardio pulmonary resuscitation (CPR) on a number of occasions. But I had never done CPR in a hospital bed.

The backboard allows for a firm foundation when CPR is performed. When CPR is administered, the chest is manually compressed using one's hands and arms. In a hospital bed during CPR, the pressure gets transferred through the body into the mattress instead of into the heart. The fact that CPR had to be performed at all spoke to the seriousness of Katie's situation, a fact that I was still discounting. There were so many people in the room between me and her I did not even see them doing it. Afterward, of course, I realized that CPR is only performed when the heart is stopping, but at the time I didn't make the connection. I was exhausted from sleep deprivation, distressed, probably in some kind of shock, and not entirely aware of everything that was happening.

Shortly after Debbie arrived, Cheryl called me on the cell phone. She was coming into Boston and needed directions. Tim took the phone and guided her right to the hospital. It was a Sunday morning and the traffic was light.

The doctors gave us an update on Katie's condition. We stared at them in disbelief. Katie had a massive lung infection that was growing rapidly. They didn't know how she got it or where, or how it settled in the lungs. This bug, as they called it, was responding to the antibiotics and was being eradicated from her bloodstream. But her lungs were filling up with blood and fluid, putting tremendous strain on her heart and other internal organs. Her little heart was overloaded and that was why her blood pressure was dropping so precipitously and so often.

Katie's heart had almost stopped three different times and rescue doses of epinephrine had been given to stimulate it. Manual compressions had been given to help the heart move back into the normal range. The challenge was the condition of the lungs, as they continued to bleed profusely. I watched the containers under the bed fill up with bloody fluid as she was suctioned by the doctors and nurses. Her chest films showed that the area of infection in the lung was growing at a rapid rate. Her right lung was completely opaque and her left lung was now partially involved. The doctors were honest with us and told us they did not know what might happen next.

6:30 a.m., Sunday, September 23:
Last Rites

At about six thirty, a short, thin lady with penetrating eyes appeared in Katie's room. She was dressed in street clothes but identified herself as Sister Carlene, a Roman Catholic sister from the hospital chaplain's unit. My mother's sister was a Dominican nun and she always dressed in her habit when she was working, so I was surprised to see a woman of the cloth without a habit. Sister Carlene already knew we were Catholic and asked me about Katie and if I thought it might be time to administer the last rites. The sacrament of the sick is one of three sacraments performed at the end of life, the others being confession and receiving holy communion. According to canon law, it may only be administered by a priest. I asked her about this and Sister Carlene told me that she was authorized to do it; in my concern for Katie, I thought it was time. She offered a prayer for healing, delivered the sacrament, and we held our hands in prayer over Katie. As she left, she told me that she would be back in a few hours to meet Cheryl, who should be there any minute, and to check on us.

With the shift change, a new team arrived to take over at seven. The night team told us that a new attending physician, the doctor in charge, would be here to explain more. At 7:02, a handsome young man wearing a white lab coat over a suit and tie bounded into the room. He introduced himself simply by his first name, Bill, "one of the doctors here." He was down to earth, a regular guy, highly energetic, and extremely interested in Katie's case. He reminded me of a swashbuckling sea captain from an old Errol Flynn movie. The most remarkable trait about him was his buoyant nature. When he smiled, and it was often, I knew he meant it. He didn't seem to have a phony bone in his body. He was real.

I was surprised that none of the doctors introduced themselves as "Doctor" So-and-So. It was always only the first name, occasionally followed by the statement "one of the doctors here." They were not pretentious. They were not impressed with themselves in the way that some doctors can be. They were working in a unit that required the highest degree of sensitivity possible for the families involved, and maybe this was one way of putting the parents and families at ease.

All of Sunday morning was a blur. Cheryl's parents arrived at seven. Cheryl got there at seven thirty and when she saw Katie, was utterly shocked. She saw all the intravenous lines and pumps, and the intubation tube in Katie's mouth, and stood there speechless.

I took Molly down to the emergency department to have her checked. The ED staff did a nasal swab on her, looking for the same germ that Katie had. In less than an hour, they determined that Molly just had a cold and was in no danger. We went back to the seventh floor and Cheryl's dad, Jim, kept Molly out in the waiting area where she could rest or play and not be underfoot, while I went back into the PICU.

I was tired and hungry. I had been awake for twenty-six hours and at last I had some family members present to help. They could listen to the medical team as reports were given, and get a feel for what was happening. I was afraid I was missing something. I still did not fully grasp all that was going on around me, though I had a front row seat. Cheryl was upset. I was upset. We still could not believe that we might lose Katie. The nurses directed us to the hospital cafeteria, so we found Molly and her grandfather and headed down to get some breakfast and coffee. After I ate, I felt much better. We hurried back to the bedside, not wanting to miss any developments. We were worried sick.

Around nine thirty, we met another day shift doctor at Katie's bedside, a tall, regal-looking man. He was about to perform a procedure that would open a cannulation site on Katie. A cannula is a small tube inserted into a vein that creates a central venous line, or CVL. A CVL gains access to a patient's bloodstream through a larger vein than one ordinarily used in an IV. Medications and blood samples are administered and taken easier with a CVL.

The tall doctor told us that an ECMO machine would use the same site, if they decided to use it. When I asked him about the ECMO machine, he seemed to think that I wouldn't understand how it worked, but he tolerated my probing questions. ECMO stood for extracorporeal membrane oxygenation, and he said that Katie might need to be placed on the ECMO machine to artificially introduce oxygen to the blood when the lungs are incapable of doing so. A large needle, or cannula, is placed directly into a large vein and circulates the blood, via a pump, into a machine. This machine has very thin filters, with the patient's blood on one side and a rich oxygen mixture on the other side. The hemoglobin in the blood attaches to the oxygen on the other side of the membrane, automatically exchanging the carbon dioxide for the oxygen and then moving on, back to the patient.

The ECMO circuit is a temporary bridge that pumps and oxygenates blood in the patient, to allow the body to heal enough to function on its own. Three to four weeks is the typical window, and after that, the circuit doesn't work very well. Blood starts to clot, oxygenation rates decline, and eventually, the organs fail and the patient dies.

I asked him how the hemoglobin knew what to do. His answer was simple but profound. He said, "It was made that way." He told me no patient's family had ever asked him these questions. I was fascinated by the concept that a machine could do some of the work that a human body could do, beyond just pumping blood. I had no idea how it worked, how it was even possible, and I wanted to learn more about it. Though distraught, anything I could learn about Katie's treatment was of interest to me.

About a year earlier, I had acquired a book at a book swap. It was a history of the Spanish flu, the worldwide influenza pandemic of 1918. I had just started to read it the week that Katie got sick. The day before she went to the hospital, I had finished the chapter on lung biology and physiology, so I was able to understand things a little better when speaking with her doctors. It was a strange occurrence after having had the book for a year, that I happened to be reading it just when the same kind of illness was ravaging my little girl.

At two thirty in the afternoon, the infectious disease, or ID, team arrived and examined Katie. With them was a group of doctors from a hospital in Philadelphia who specialized in the study of the human lung. They had flown up that morning for a brief stay, and were eager to examine Katie, because her case was so rare. They introduced themselves to us, and the first thing they asked was whether we had any chickens or pet birds in the house, just as the lead doctor in the emergency department had the night before. We told them no. They then asked if there were any old buildings on our property that used to have chickens living in them where the children might have played. Again, the answer was no.

I thought it was interesting that the first question from the ED doctors, and now the ID team, would center on chickens. We had chickens when I was a kid, and I got sick of dealing with them early in life, so we never had them at our house. I wondered what the connection was, what they were looking for. They told us the same thing, that sometimes chickens carry diseases that can cause symptoms similar to what Katie had. A doctor friend of mine says that chickens are known to cause a fungal disease called aspergillosis, but these doctors mentioned a bacterial disease that they were worried about. That means it was more likely they were worried about psittacosis, an unusual disease caused by a bacteria called chlamydia (not the same as the sexually transmitted kind). It is most common in parrots, parakeets, pigeons, and doves, and only rarely occurs in chickens.

During the afternoon, the nurses suggested that Cheryl and I should go to the families' office to get a room in the parent sleep quarters. Katie was stable and Cheryl's parents were entertaining Molly, so we went downstairs to find the place. The people there gave us a room and a key and we went off to find our new temporary home. It was located in another building attached to the main hospital and was quiet and out of the way. No television and no refrigerator offering five-dollar beer, but it would do. We weren't able to consider sleeping yet, so we hurried back to Katie's bedside.

It was now near three and we decided that Molly should go home with her grandparents to North Attleboro, Massachusetts, as the hospital was no place for a two-year-old. She'd missed her nap that day and was getting sleepy and cranky. She loved her grandmother and was not upset about going with her and Jim. They left and we went down to the cafeteria to get something to eat. I had now been awake for thirty-six hours.

Throughout the afternoon we had been briefed by the doctors on Katie's status and what was happening with her. I called my mother frequently to keep her updated. She was worrying about two of her children now; my sister was in Lebanon, New Hampshire, beside her forty-three-year-old husband who was dying from leukemia, and us in Boston. She was also caring for her eleven-year-old granddaughter, my sister's daughter. All of this was stressful for her—she was anxious and fraught with worry about all the terrible sicknesses the family faced.

We met a new doctor late in the afternoon, who was the attending physician for the next shift. Trim, impeccably dressed under his lab coat, with well-shined dress shoes, Connor (another "one of the doctors here") was cool, reserved, and handsome. He had the calculating eyes of a gunfighter, the presence of an executive, and the poise of a fencing expert. He reminded me of my old fencing instructor. Polite and intelligent, he was quiet, but not because he was unsure or afraid. He was clearly thinking about Katie's options, trying to figure out the best course of action. Later, as the days drew on, after the rounds were done and the team had moved on to their other duties, he would return to the same spot outside of Katie's room and strike the same pose: his left arm crossed on his chest and his right elbow cradled in his left hand, with his right fist resting on his chin, searching his mind for a solution to her sickness.

10:00 p.m., Sunday, September 23:
Second Pneumothorax and Chest Tube

At ten Sunday night the team decided to place another chest tube into Katie's right side to drain some of the fluid that was building up inside of her. Katie's right lung had developed another pneumothorax, and the tall, regal-looking doctor performed the procedure between her fifth and sixth ribs, getting a gush of air and almost a pint of serous fluid, the translucent yellow fluid found throughout the body cavity. He stitched it up and her condition was stable for now.

Dr. Connor and the buoyant day shift doctor, Bill, had been talking all afternoon about the ECMO option, and started asking us what we thought about it. I told them that I understood it to mean that Katie's condition was getting worse. We assured them that we supported whatever decision they made. We didn't really understand any of it and were grossly unqualified to comment. And we were running out of options.

I was too tired to be of any help to anybody. At around eleven we decided to go to the parent sleep quarters and get some rest. Katie appeared to be stable after the second chest tube was placed and it was time for me to get some sleep. We had just made it into bed when the phone rang. It was the computer nurse I had met the night before. She told me that we needed to come back immediately, since Katie was very sick, and the nurses felt we should be there. Katie had been sick all day, so I wondered if it was just because she had come in at the shift change and hadn't seen Katie earlier. "How sick is she?" I asked.

The nurse said, "She can't get any sicker. Get over here now."

We put our clothes back on and ran over to seven south and up to Katie's room. She had coded again and the doctors had decided to put her on ECMO or she was going to die.

With ECMO preparations came another doctor, a vascular surgeon: a short, energetic man dressed in scrubs with a mask around his neck. He passed me one of his cards as he explained what was involved with ECMO and said I could call him anytime if I had questions. He presented no more concern about performing another cannulation procedure on Katie's jugular vein than if he were loading his dishwasher at home. He put us at ease with his confident and cheerful manner. After a nearly two-hour procedure, Katie was placed on ECMO, and things began to stabilize immediately. How a man can be that upbeat and positive at one o'clock in the morning in a pediatric intensive care unit is a marvel to me. He must love his job.

At two in the morning—it was now Monday, September 24—we again retired to the parent sleep quarters. I had now been awake for forty-five hours, and I collapsed into bed.

Later that same day, day three of Katie's admission, we found that the ECMO circuit had bought us some time. Katie stabilized as soon as it was functioning. Her blood pressure evened out, and her blood gas readings improved. Gone were the wild swings in blood pressure, the code blues, the frantic CPR, and the sense of emergency and imminent death. Everything seemed to be going well. After twenty-four hours of tension, fear, and worry, ECMO offered us welcome relief.

I had a chance to appreciate what was being done for Katie. She was being monitored for heart and lung function, kidney function, and blood gases, all together telling the team what Katie's body was doing and how it was reacting to the medication. Katie had sixteen infusion pumps attached to her veins, each pumping a different medication. There were two people at her bedside at all times, a highly trained intensive care unit nurse and a nurse ECMO specialist who ran and monitored the machine. Doctors and nurses would come and go all the time, checking on her and on us. It truly was an intensive care environment.

Never once did anyone do or say anything to offend us or make us feel uncomfortable. Every person we talked to was eager to explain what was going on and seemed genuinely interested in and concerned for Katie and for us. They were all intelligent. I once commented to Dr. Connor about the high quality of the staff I met in the PICU. His response was, "There are no idiots in the ICU."

After Katie had stabilized, I asked Dr. Bill what he thought about things at that time. He told me there was cause for encouragement and that ECMO had bought us some time, but he qualified it with a comment drawn from his years of experience. He reminded me of the still-present danger by saying, "We have never had a ship sail so far from home and come back."

I'd gotten some sleep the night before; it was the longest time I had ever gone without sleep in my life. I had pulled a twenty-four-hour shift many times in the past while plowing snow, but this time was almost twice that. The stress of seeing Katie in such a condition made it all the more exhausting. Cheryl slept about the same amount of time as I did, close to six hours, but it was a fitful sleep for both of us.

As soon as we woke up, we headed for Katie's bedside. Nothing like this had ever happened to us; we had no benchmarks by which to judge the situation. It was exhausting and terrifying. Cheryl and I talked to each other all the time, trying to get a handle on what we were seeing unfold. We were still able to function, but in my view, we were not functioning very well. There was nothing we could do; the whole affair was out of our hands. All we could do was watch as things developed. We didn't cry, we didn't suffer any emotional breakdowns, although admittedly, this was the kind of event that can cause a breakdown to happen. We had to accept our fate, and Katie's fate, come what may. We still had Molly to care for, too. This was the time in a marriage when it really mattered whom we chose for a partner. When things go bad, we need to be able to draw on our reserves of inner strength and support the other person. Unknown to us at the time, our inner strength had also become each other's strength.

At eight thirty that morning I called Katie's preschool to tell them about her condition, so that they could be on the lookout for students with similar symptoms. I spoke with the school nurse and she told me she would call all the students who were absent that day to check on their status.

I started thinking about bird droppings now that two different doctors had asked me about them. I recalled that one day at Katie's daycare, I noticed a mourning dove nest in the ceiling of the alcove at the entrance. Katie would sometimes sit on the top step while waiting for the bus to pick her up and take her to preschool. I wondered if she might have put her hand in the microscopic remains of the droppings and been exposed that way. I called my longtime friend who worked at the agency that owned the building. I told her what was going on and suggested she get a cleaning crew over there right then with a pressure washer to clean the steps and blast the doves out of their nest, young and all. She was as stunned about this turn of events as any of us and agreed to do it as soon as she could get some people over there. If that was where Katie was exposed, we both wanted to prevent any other children from getting the same sickness.

CHAPTER 6

A Dubious Reprieve

Once Katie was hooked up to the ECMO machine, her course started to become less worrisome. Katie had time to heal and the medical team had time to monitor and assess her condition. Several days passed, each one more or less like the previous one. She was moved just down the hall to a bigger room in the PICU. We looked for small signs of improvement, and the doctors reading the reports hourly or more often watched for the signs that would indicate that she would pull out of it.

It became a grueling vigil of waiting for me and Cheryl, and for all of us. We were lost when we talked about medicine with the doctors. They were patient with us, spending lots of time decoding the data and explaining it in terms we could understand. They were wonderful. A young female resident, Dr. Ashley, took extra time with us, returning to Katie's bedside after rounds were done to explain every aspect of Katie's course. She took an interest in us and Katie, even telling us where to find the best ice cream shop in the neighborhood, when we needed a break from the serious atmosphere found in the hospital room. Dr. Bill called my mother regularly to give her reports in medical terms. My mother understood them better than we did. She also seemed to know what was coming, because of her years as a nurse.

Monday also brought a new day shift social worker, Miss Stevens, assigned to us by the hospital. She was eager and helpful, and I suspect she was watching us for signs of psychological abnormalities. She later commented to me that she thought we were strong people and a mutually committed couple. I responded with a line from John Milton's *Paradise Lost* that I had memorized years before: "To be weak is miserable, doing or suffering." To my great surprise, she knew the author and knew the quote. It marks one of the few times in my life that I have quoted a bit of literature when the receiving party knew what I was talking about. It was refreshing and made my day. I studied classic literature in high school and college, and I still read voraciously. If I remember a quote that fits the situation at hand, I sometimes repeat it out loud.

Cheryl and I took this time to regroup and figure out what we could do. We had both left New Hampshire in a rush and left a lot hanging. We took turns going back to our house to take care of some pressing housekeeping issues. Cheryl went home and got some clean clothes and our overnight bags, and stopped at her office to inform them about what was happening.

Just two weeks before Katie got sick, Cheryl's boss at the government agency where she worked had told her that her annual employment contract would not be renewed, and would end in six months. She had been a federal wildlife biologist for thirteen years, ten of them at her current office. Her contract had to be renewed every year, and since this was year ten, her boss either had to make her a permanent employee, or get rid of her. Because of her annual raises and a few grade promotions, she was making reasonably good money and carrying the health insurance for our family. She was an expensive employee. If her contract was not renewed, her boss could hire a recent college graduate for a lot less money. Such is the risk of working under employment-at-will contracts.

To the agency her position was a line item on a budget spreadsheet. But to Cheryl, her position was also her identity. She held a bachelor's and a master's degree in wildlife biology, six years' worth of college education and thirteen years' experience in the field. Even with her education and experience, she was still not a permanent employee. Despite our personal tragedy, her contract was not renewed, and her career was over, at the worst possible time in her life.

In the federal employment system, employees can ask other federal employees to donate their unused leave time in an emergency. Cheryl applied for this benefit and received enough donated leave time to pay her salary through the end of her contract, which expired in April of the next year. It was a big help to us. Later we found out that Cheryl received more than five years' worth of donated leave time from other federal employees, a resounding testament to the generosity of those on the federal payroll.

Our friends came to visit us and Katie, and some of them wanted to take us out to eat. There was an Irish pub near the hospital and we would occasionally walk over there for a time out, soaking up the warm fall sunshine. It was therapeutic to get off campus and outside, if only for a short time. Katie was always foremost in our thoughts.

By now most of our friends had heard about what was happening. They all wanted to help in some way, so I encouraged them to come to the hospital and give blood. Katie was using a lot of blood while on the ECMO circuit and new blood was needed all the time. She would eventually use more than 260 units. The need for blood in a hospital is chronic. Katie's blood type was A positive, but more than one time during her stay I noticed that the blood going into the ECMO machine was O, not A positive. I surmised that this meant that the blood bank was out of her blood type and had to default to the universal donor type. This concerned me greatly and I talked with the blood collection office, and we discussed what to do about it. They offered to conduct a blood drive in Katie's name. I knew if they could get to our area in New Hampshire, we could fill a blood collection bus every day for weeks.

However, there were problems with insurance and licensing in New Hampshire, and also with the time and distance involved in transporting the blood that far. I told them I had friends who were helicopter pilots, and their companies and government agencies had offered to pick up the blood in New Hampshire and fly it to Boston free of charge, if that would aid in collection and timeliness. The insurmountable problem was one of licensing. The nurses who worked in the blood collection bus were not licensed in New Hampshire. To become licensed would have taken far too long. We needed to find a place in Massachusetts to conduct a blood drive.

The blood collection office suggested that churches were historically a good place to have blood drives, so we approached the parish where we were married and where Katie was baptized. They readily agreed and we scheduled a blood drive for late October. We have conducted a blood drive at this church two or three times a year ever since, in April and October, and sometimes in January. It has proven to be one of the best blood drives for the hospital, bringing in between fifty and seventy units each time. We have conducted twenty-nine blood drives and collected almost fifteen hundred units of blood. As good as that number sounds, in total, it is still in the single-digit percentages of the total amount of blood the hospital uses in one year.

It is hard to articulate how terrifying it is to have a child in a pediatric intensive care unit who needs blood transfusions to stay alive, and to know that this child's blood type is in short supply, or worse, unavailable. That didn't happen to us, but it has happened. I have a new respect for those who donate blood. I hope the reader will consider donating blood, and especially platelets, directly to the nearest hospital as often as possible.

Katie's doctors were anxious to wean her off the ECMO circuit and other machines. One of these was called a continuous positive airway pressure machine, or CPAP. This machine inserted air into her lungs to keep them open and to assist her with breathing. It was used in conjunction with a high-frequency oscillation ventilator, or Hi-Fi, a machine that moves gases into and out of the artificially inflated lungs. If her lungs improved to the point where she could breathe on her own, she could be slowly disconnected from the artificial breathing machines and eventually taken off the ECMO.

Occasionally they would back off the settings on the machines and monitor her blood gases to see if any lung function was returning. Initially the signs were encouraging.

Cheryl and I stayed at her bedside. We often talked to Katie, in the hope that she could hear us. With all the medication she was receiving, it would theoretically be impossible for her to respond to us. However, when Cheryl or I told Katie that we were leaving the room to go for lunch or to leave for the evening, we would notice a spike in her heart rate. It was just like her to become anxious when we had to be apart. It seemed to me that she could hear us, but we will never know for sure. I can't explain the change in the heart rate that we saw on her monitors.

We discussed Katie's case with the team every day. Dr. Connor told me that there were few cases in medical history to compare with Katie's. He could find only six others, a confirmation of the rarity of her sickness. The infectious disease team had identified the germ as MRSA, of which there were seventy-three known types. Katie's was in the lungs, which was what made it so dangerous. As it was explained to me later, necrotizing pneumonia destroys the cells in the alveoli in the lung. White blood cells attack the MRSA germ at the cellular level and die in the process, creating a crust over the membrane that exchanges the oxygen and carbon dioxide, CO_2, blocking all gas transfer. Significantly, the detritus also prevents antibiotics from entering and attacking the germ. It was a numbers game—the more alveolar cells that were damaged irreparably, the less oxygen could be exchanged, and the less antibiotic could be delivered.

On September 29, day seven of her stay, the team gave her a wake-up test. The medications used to keep her sedated and paralyzed were gradually withdrawn, allowing her to briefly wake up and look around. On this day Katie opened her eyes, looked around, and moved all four of her limbs. She was quickly remedicated, but it gave us hope that she was able to wake up. It was encouraging. There wasn't much Cheryl and I could do. We stayed with Katie as much as we could, talking to her and reading her favorite stories. Except for the spike in her heartrate when we told her we were leaving, there was no response.

The next day the team ordered a bronchoscopy, a procedure that allows the doctor to enter the airway with special tools and physically remove any obstructions, such as blood clots, that might be impeding air flow to the lungs. This was performed by a lovely young female doctor with sad eyes. She could tell that Katie's prognosis was not a good one and though she tried to be chipper, her face gave away her feelings. She removed a large blood clot from Katie's airway, which gave us hope, but at the same time, reminded us of just how sick Katie was.

The Pigeon

Katie's new room in the PICU was much bigger than the first one. The windows, like all the windows there, offered a partial view of the city skyline. The view was cut up by other tall buildings, and directly outside her window was the roof of a lower building that was attached to the hospital. There were a few mechanical apparatuses located on that roof, and catwalks and handrails that allowed access for maintenance. As in most cities, pigeons congregated in those areas.

Every day as I looked out the window, I saw pigeons coming and going about their pigeon business. But there was one pigeon in particular that always seemed to be there. He never flew away, he never ate; he just paced up and down the catwalk right outside the window to her room. When I was a child, we kept tumbler and fantail pigeons as livestock and I learned their habits by being around them all the time. I also learned to identify different birds by observing their plumage. Often this is the only way to tell which bird is which. This pigeon had distinctive markings that made it easy to identify: a bright purple neck and little black stripes on the wings. Cheryl identified him, too. She has an eye for bird markings, being a wildlife biologist, and her first master's degree was in ornithological statistics. She knows birds.

This bird was there every day, all day. I began to wonder what he was up to, walking back and forth, looking directly into the room. He would walk by in one direction looking in, turn around, and walk back the other way, turning his head to look in again. This went on for hours, all day long, day after day.

I was under extreme stress at the time, with Katie so sick, and the longer it went on without her getting much better, the more it looked to us like she might not recover. I began to get paranoid about this animal. After all the talk and questions about bird droppings in the first few hours of Katie's admission, I was terrified of that bird. Pigeons are extremely dirty animals and their droppings in any quantity are hazardous to humans.

The windows are hermetically sealed, as is the entire floor, and cannot be opened. Air exchangers and purifiers occupy two entire floors of the building, cleansing the air for the patients. There was no way his pigeon germs could get at my baby, though he was only a few feet away. Still, he was giving me the creeps and I wanted to kill him. It would be so easy to exterminate that pigeon—if I could get to him.

I began to have thoughts of doing things found in horror movies. I thought this pigeon was some diabolical entity, possessed by the devil, or maybe was the devil, waiting for my Katie girl to die so he could claim her soul. I wanted to find the entry to the catwalk, climb out on the ledge that was seven stories high, lunge at this bird, and snap his neck. I had thoughts of grabbing a chair, throwing it through the window, and jumping on this evil creature before it could get away.

I thought of bringing a shotgun to the hospital so I could stand in the courtyard and shoot every pigeon that I could before the police came and took me away. I had visions of me being caught with a net, forced into a straitjacket, and loaded into an ambulance, kicking and screaming and ranting about the devil in the form of a pigeon that was trying to usher my Katie into the netherworld. That was a story the television stations would love. Thankfully, good breeding and education prevented me from acting on my primal impulses. My friend Mason thinks that the pigeon was angelic and not diabolic, that it was Katie's heavenly escort, so he is glad I didn't kill it. I will never forget that pigeon and I still wonder what was going on. It was very unusual behavior for a pigeon.

Time in the PICU ground on. Cheryl had been going home to her parents' house in North Attleboro every few days to visit with Molly and to get a good night's sleep. I went with her on the evening of Tuesday, October 2, and while we were gone, Katie was given another wake-up test. We wanted to be there so she could see us, but it was done in the morning on Wednesday before we arrived back at the hospital. Katie's nurse told us that once again she opened her eyes, looked around, and moved all four of her limbs. "She's in there," she said.

On Thursday, October 4, I returned to our house in New Hampshire to take care of some pressing business. While there I took time to go see my primary care physician. I told him I was having a lot of stress, and he prescribed me some pills to help me relax and get some sleep. I have never been a fan of drugs and this time was no different. I took two doses, 12 hours apart, but they didn't seem to do much of anything for me. Katie was still sick and not getting better, and he couldn't prescribe medication to fix that. I drove back to the hospital that night.

Katie had been in bed, immobilized, for nearly two weeks. One of the things that begins to happen to patients in this condition is called "foot drop," a condition where the foot literally begins to droop from inactivity. This can be corrected with a splint, which holds the foot at a nearly right angle to the leg.

One day a man came in to Katie's room with two splints and attached them to her feet. He asked me to sign a form and then presented me with a bill for two thousand dollars. He told me that it may not be covered by our health insurance, so the amount was payable upon delivery. He stood there and looked me, judging my reaction, as though he were expecting me to write him a check.

I calmly told him to take the splints off Katie, if he was that worried about the bill. He apologized for asking and left immediately. This was the only time during our stay that I had any mildly negative interaction with anyone at the hospital, and it was just business, nothing more. In fairness to the splint man, he did not know our story or what was wrong with Katie, and it is standard procedure in some allied medical practices to ask for payment upon delivery. The practice he worked for was independent of the hospital and had probably been burned by insurance companies in the past. He was polite and clearly uneasy about posing the question, but he did his duty and got out of there fast. I respect his professional approach to a difficult subject and his courage in doing his job.

On Saturday, October 6, Molly's godmother, Xander, flew up from Washington, DC, to visit us. She is a family friend and was living at our house when Katie was born. At the time, she had just returned from a year abroad on a Fulbright study, and needed time to find a new place to live. She is a lawyer now and had just started her first job at a law firm in early September. Katie and Molly had been the flower girls at her wedding at the Rollins Chapel at Dartmouth College just three weeks before, on Labor Day weekend. She was troubled to see Katie in that condition. What a terrible way for her and her husband to start their marriage. She was strong, visiting Katie in the PICU for most of the day and offering what moral support to us that she could muster. We were glad she made the time to come up and see Katie.

Every day at three in the afternoon, a man with penetrating, intelligent eyes would come through the PICU with a floor cleaner. There was a dignity about him that transcended his position. Some of the staff disliked him because he would come through with that noisy floor scrubber no matter what was going on, moving wheeled carts and laundry baskets and shooing nurses out of the way. I had worked summers at my high school cleaning and waxing the hallways and gymnasium floors twenty-five years ago. The machine he used was more advanced than the ones I had used. It was high tech.

One day I asked him about it, how it worked, and if he would mind showing it to me. Without hesitation he shut it off, opened the hood, and proceeded to tell me everything about it. He was proud of his work and delighted that someone took an interest in it. He knew that machine as well as any technician, explaining things to me in technical terms that I did not understand. This man was a floor professional. He was not stupid; in fact, his intelligence was striking. He knew exactly what the machine did, knew exactly what was required to get a perfect finish every time. I was impressed. He was far more than a simple janitor; he was confident and secure, eager to explain in articulate terms what it was that he did. I was glad I took the time to meet this man. In less than five minutes, he gave me a small distraction from the slow-motion terror we were facing with Katie's illness.

I passed him on the street outside the hospital about a year later when I was there to give blood. He did not recognize me and I did not stop to speak to him. The look on his face was that of a serious, sober gentleman, and I wondered to myself if he might be a guardian angel masquerading as a janitor. If we are to find guardian angels in this life, I submit that they would be drawn to a place such as this hospital. Maybe I'm superstitious, but it wouldn't hurt to have a few undercover angels on the staff.

CHAPTER 7

Losing the Fight

That Sunday, October 7, we learned that the chest films showed that Katie's progress was not good. The doctors were openly concerned and communicated their fears to us. Several bronchoscopies had been completed but had not delivered the results they were hoping to see. Though some blood clots had been removed, her lung function was still getting worse. The X-rays indicated that something was covering both lungs, which they thought were blood clots. They couldn't really tell what it was.

That night we both went to North Attleboro to visit Molly. Cheryl's mother had called to tell us that Molly missed us and wanted to see us. Before we could return to the hospital on Monday morning, Katie developed yet another pneumothorax and required yet another chest tube. It was an ominous sign.

There was nothing we could do when such things happened, but to be absent made it all the worse. Our fears of being absent if something went wrong were with us all the time, a modern Sword of Damocles in a medical setting. We had to juggle our concern for Katie with our responsibilities to Molly. Molly missed us. Her life was as disrupted as any of ours, but she was too young to comprehend. There was little we could do for Katie except stand at her bedside and pray she would recover. I still think she could hear us and knew we were there.

On Monday, October 8, Dr. Connor, the attending physician, expressed grave concern about the lack of progress. He felt that something was very wrong and was concerned that Katie's lungs might not recover before the ECMO started to develop problems. He ordered a CT scan, short for computed tomography, a high-resolution X-ray of her lungs, to see if it could determine what was wrong. This involved moving Katie out of the PICU and down to radiology, a risky venture with such a critically ill patient. While she was being moved, her vital signs showed great distress, but she got through it, and the procedure gave the team more information about what might be going on with Katie's lungs. We wouldn't know what they found until the next day.

Later that day, when the rounds were done and Dr. Connor returned to check on us, I asked him about Katie's course. Cheryl and I talked about it, and it appeared to us that Katie was losing the fight. We didn't want to prolong her suffering. She had been through so much; we wondered how much more her little body could take.

Specifically, I asked the doctor how to know when it was time to end the fight. I told him I was concerned about all the time and money involved. I knew we had good health insurance, but I also knew there were lifetime caps on coverage, and I didn't know what would happen when those caps were met. I wondered if the hospital would have to withdraw treatment, or what. I was also concerned that since it looked like Katie was not going to make it, why we should prolong the effort.

Dr. Connor's response was authoritative and quick, almost curt, allowing a tiny glimpse of his frustration: "We don't care about the time, and we don't care about the money. It is expensive and it is time consuming, but if we can save her life, we are going to do it." My question was answered and dismissed in two sentences.

My friend and former co-worker, Tina, came to visit us the next day and gave me a ride home that afternoon so I could get more clean clothes. On the way home I stopped at Cheryl's office to drop off some paperwork for her. While I was there, I received a call from the hospital. They needed authorization to perform surgery on Katie and couldn't locate Cheryl on the hospital campus. (She later told me she was eating lunch in the cafeteria, which is located in the cellar of the hospital, and had no cell phone service.) While I was gone, Dr. Connor had decided to perform exploratory surgery on Katie's lungs. The CT scan from the previous day had revealed a mass over her lungs that could not be identified without opening the chest. The team thought it might be a massive blood clot preventing the lungs from returning to normal. Though risky, surgery was the only way to determine what was wrong inside Katie's chest. I gave the authorization and hurried back to my house to gather our clean clothes and hitch a ride back to Boston. My father and brother came to pick me up and we headed south in Dad's minivan.

While we were on the road, Cheryl called me at about one thirty to tell me that Katie was going in for surgery at three, and for me to hurry. She was able to get a priest to administer the sacrament of the sick, which he did at one, before the surgery. This had been a concern for us as there was some doubt in our minds about Sister Carlene's authority to perform last rites. Canon law is clear that it must be performed by a priest, and now it was done.

I kept thinking to myself that October 10 was the day my grandmother died, thirty years ago to the day, and it was comforting to think that she was watching and praying for our Katie girl.

We got to the hospital just before Katie was wheeled into surgery. Dad and Chris got to see her go. They waited with us for her to come out and to get the report from the surgeon. At five the surgeon came to see us in the waiting room. He was concise and to the point, speaking in precise medical terms about exactly what it was that he found. He said, "It was very difficult," a phrase he repeated three times in the few minutes he spent with us. He told us that the bleeding was profuse, that they couldn't stop it, and in fact, that they did not sew Katie up. He had packed the wound to try to stop the bleeding and was afraid that if he sutured her closed, the chest cavity would fill with blood. He said Katie did not take the surgery well, her blood pressure had dropped dramatically, and he felt that it was very hard on her body.

His body language and the look on his face said it all. It was over. He never said it that way, but I could tell from the way he was describing

Katie's condition there was nothing more that could be done. He shook hands with all of us and patted me on the back. I could see in his eyes his genuine concern for Katie and for us. He told us we could get a more detailed report from Dr. Connor when we saw him in the PICU the next day.

That evening Katie's pediatrician, Chris, in New Hampshire, called me to ask how things were going. I told him things did not look good. I told him about the surgery and what the surgeon had told us. He offered what support he could and we hung up. He must have known we were nearing the end of the fight. Cheryl and I could see it, we lived it every day, and we knew it would be over soon. The sense of impending doom was everywhere in our minds. It was overpowering.

There was nothing we could do about Katie's sickness. Cheryl and I talked throughout the crisis, and we both knew the end was here. We didn't want to see her go on in such a state, and now it was clear there was no hope of recovery. We were honest with each other, and the medical team was honest with us. The news came as macabre relief, knowing that her suffering would soon be over, but it also came with the realization that we were going to lose Katie. It was a difficult trade, and I didn't think we were ready, but we were as ready as we could be. I was incredulous that with all this technology and the best medical staff in the world, there was no more to be done.

The next day, October 11, Thursday, we saw Dr. Connor at ten o'clock in the morning. He confirmed what we already knew: Katie's prognosis wasn't sound. Though Katie had been on life support for all but a few minutes of her stay in Boston, that support could no longer save her life. She was barely hanging on. He suggested we have a meeting with the medical team at four in the PICU conference room to review our options. Jim and Ann came to the hospital with Molly to hear things firsthand.

At four we assembled in the conference room with Dr. Bill, Dr. Connor, and others: Miss Stevens, the social worker, Sister Carlene, and our family friend, Sande, who was visiting for the day and tended to Molly during the meeting. The very presence of the social worker and the sister was evidence of what was coming. Dr. Connor told us there were three options, all of them bad. The surgeon's report showed that the right lung was entirely necrotic tissue, and significant portions of the left lung were now also necrotic. He had looked at the tissue under the microscope and found only diseased tissue, and in some cases, no tissue at all, only pustules. The right lung was dead, and there was not enough tissue in the left lung to support life. ECMO was beginning to clot, and the CT scan showed that she had bleeding in her brain.

There were three options.

1. Do nothing and eventually ECMO would clot and shut down.
2. Stop ECMO and see if the left lung could support life with the ventilator.
3. Withdraw treatment and shut everything down.

He closed his presentation with the words, "I couldn't be sorrier." It was clear that he meant it.

I asked about the possibility of a lung transplant, if healthy lungs could be found to replace Katie's diseased ones. He told us they had tried that in the past, but because of the blood thinners required for the ECMO circuit to work, the patient would bleed to death before the transplanted lungs could heal. In addition, the MRSA infection was still raging, and it was likely that healthy lungs would be infected during the operation, creating the same problem Katie was currently facing. Because of this, Katie was not a candidate for a lung transplant. The bad news we had feared most had arrived. It was over.

In the PICU, twelve-hour shifts are the standard workday. On this day, one nurse who had taken a special liking to us was working and knew the end was near. She volunteered to stay over on her shift, which ended at seven in the evening, so she could be the one with Katie and us at the end. I could tell it upset her but she wanted to do it, exhibiting a strong and professional presence right to the finish.

We chose option three, to be instituted later that day. Dr. Connor suggested we call my mother for one last visit. She arrived about 8:50 p.m. with Dad and Chris. She knelt and said a prayer and they all said goodbye and left. The doctors stopped the paralytic Katie was receiving in the event that she might open her eyes one last time. She didn't; all we saw was a little twitching of her tongue.

The nurse set up a bed next to Katie so Cheryl could lie down beside her and read her some stories, all her favorites. The nurse made a cast of her hand and took prints of her hands and feet. She also cut five locks of Katie's hair for us to keep. That evening I kept remembering that October 11 was the anniversary of the Battle of Valcour Island in Lake Champlain, fought during the American Revolution, a battle the American side lost. I knew we had lost this fight, too.

Doctors and nurses see a lot of patients with severe illnesses and, over time, become somewhat necessarily inured to tragedy. A doctor friend of mine, who is on the admissions committee of a major medical school, says they look for extremely empathetic applicants to be doctors, knowing that repeated exposure to tragedy will predictably decrease their empathy, hoping they will end up as doctors with the right balance of empathy and emotional distance. This is so they can both relate to patients and families as empathetic caregivers and still have enough emotional distance to keep doing their job for decades.

When the time came to withdraw treatment, it was anticlimactic. Fifty-five minutes into Friday morning, Katie's nurse administered an additional dose of morphine, and the nurse ECMO specialist, who was crying, simply placed a clamp on the line that pumped the blood through Katie's body. That was it. No plug was pulled; her life blood was literally clamped off while we waited for her heart to stop. The night shift attending physician, another tall man with fierce and intelligent eyes, watched the monitors as her heart rate declined rapidly. It was evidence of just how much life support Katie required. As soon as the meds were stopped, her heart rate plummeted. In just four minutes from the time that treatment was withdrawn, it was over. Katie died at fifty-nine minutes after midnight on Friday, October 12.

We were right beside her while she died. After the doctor pronounced her, we stayed with her for a few minutes. Then Katie's nurse offered to walk us out to the waiting room where we were to meet the doctor for a consultation. She told us she would need a few minutes to clean Katie up, then we could come back and see her one last time. We walked out of the PICU and headed for the waiting room in a heavy daze. At last, it was over. The enormity of our loss began to dawn on us. It was overwhelming.

Though we had lost the fight, there was a sense of relief knowing that Katie's suffering was done. I called my mother from the waiting room to tell her Katie was gone. She said there had been a tremendous lightning flash a few minutes ago, a flash that stayed lit up, not intermittent, with thunder, but no rain. She took that as a sign from Katie. My brother saw it too, and thought the thunder was Katie laughing. I called our friend Sande, who also reported a strange light in the sky. None of us can remember the last time there was a thunderstorm in October in New Hampshire.

We sat together for a short time when two doctors came in to go over things with us. The first doctor expressed his condolences in a compassionate way and tried to comfort us as best he could. The first thing he asked us about was whether we would permit an autopsy on Katie's body. He said the hospital wanted to learn everything they could about her illness, and a postmortem would help to advance science. We heartily endorsed the idea of an autopsy, and in my ignorance, I said, "Take the lungs and put them in a jar, so other doctors can see them."

Politely he said, "We don't do that anymore. We just take a sample for the microscope." Cheryl and I both believed we had a duty to humanity to allow her case to be studied in any way that could benefit the next family in our position. We had to sign a release form and a few other forms, and they left us with more sincere condolences. Soon afterward, Katie's nurse came back and brought us in to see her for the last time. She was clean and comfy, all tucked into her hospital bed. The IVs were out of her arms and the CPAP and intubation tube were gone. She looked at peace.

What I noticed most was how quiet it was in her room. No monitors and pumps running, the ECMO not circulating her blood, the oxygen machine turned off and quiet. The lights were still turned down low. Finally, like us, Katie looked relieved. I said a prayer quietly to myself and wished her good luck on her way to heaven. Oddly, perhaps, we were not crying. I don't know if it was because we had known it was coming and had plenty of time to prepare ourselves, or if we were in shock, or if we were just too drained emotionally to muster the tears. Cheryl is emotionally strong, and if ever there were a time when that mattered, it was now. We said our final goodbyes to our Katie girl and walked out of the PICU for the last time. Except for the other patients behind the curtains in their rooms, there was not a soul to be seen as we walked out the back way of Seven South. It was a cold and brutally lonely spot at that moment in time.

We made our way back to the parent sleep quarters and into bed. We slept, or rather, rested fitfully, until seven in the morning, when we got up and gathered our things together. We brought our room key back to the office for families and relayed the terrible news to the staff. Everyone just stared at us in silence. The look on their faces said it all. I'm sure they had heard this kind of news countless times before, but each time is different, each time represents a new tragedy. Our lives had been changed forever.

CHAPTER 8

Devastated

On Friday morning, October 12, we drove from Boston to Cheryl's parents' house in North Attleboro, observing the morning traffic pour into the city, watching so many people going about their business. For them, nothing had happened, nothing had changed. But our world as we knew it had ended. We drove on, mostly in silence, without crying or even really talking about what we had been through. We got to Cheryl's parents' house at ten. Molly was so happy to see us that it made us forget the tragedy for a minute, but only for a minute. I felt lost, totally adrift. I had no energy or desire to do anything. I found a beer in the fridge and sat down in the living room to gather my thoughts while Molly sat on my lap. She told me all about her grandparents' kitties and how much fun she had playing with them. In the egocentric world of a two-year-old, it was just another day, and at last Mum and Dad were home. She never asked about Katie.

It was a mild day, so Molly and I went out in the yard to play. We ran around the lawn just like we always did, but everything I did felt mechanical, missing some key part. We fooled around most of the day, dreading what was to come next in our lives. Jim and Ann didn't say much, as there wasn't much to say. Ann cried all day, but Cheryl and I didn't. We were too numb to do much of anything. Jim cooked dinner and made extra, to send us home with some food. Ann made cookies. It was a struggle to eat anything.

We stayed in North Attleboro that night, trying to understand what we had been through. The darkest days of our lives were now hard upon us. I wasn't sure what would happen next. It felt like a huge burden had been lifted from us, in exchange for another, more repressive load. We were relieved of the stress and worry about Katie and what would happen to her. The realization that we had lost her presented new problems. I have read about the five stages of grief, and I never really felt it could be so easily and neatly catalogued. It is overwhelming, all encompassing, fills every thought in one's mind. Everything had changed violently in a different direction. We still had Molly to care for, so there was a semblance of normalcy retained. She didn't understand what had happened, and we had to keep her life as normal as possible while trying to process the loss of her sister.

I had heard and read stories about families being destroyed by the loss of a child. Many are not able to handle the stress and adapt to the changes. I didn't know if we could, either. Everything was on the table.

At four that afternoon, we packed up the car with Molly's things and lots of food and flowers and finally got on the road, headed for home. One of the strangest feelings I have ever experienced was driving that car with Katie's empty car seat in the back. The finality of her death really hit me hard for the first time, and I cried all the way home. Somehow, we made it, and when we walked in the front door, Cheryl and I both felt that Katie was in the house waiting for us. We felt her presence everywhere. It made me feel comfortable. I could almost hear her laughter and giggles, but the presence I felt was not that of a little girl. The feeling I sensed was that of a liberated soul, a mature and effusive spirit. This was important to me because I feared that it would be unbearable to be in our house with her gone. But it was not unbearable, it was comforting.

We found the house not at all like we had left it. There was food everywhere. On the kitchen table there was a note from my old friend, Sister Leona, a nun from the church I attended in my youth and young adulthood. My brother and I had served as altar boys there. We started attending Mass at a different parish that was much closer, in Franklin, the next town over, and I never saw her anymore. I had not heard about her for twenty years. As it turned out, she had been working in Franklin for some time, though we didn't know it. There on my kitchen table was a note from her telling me she had found me once again and was here to help.

When she heard about our situation, she took the time to drive over to my town and knocked on doors until she found out where I lived, which is no easy task. I live out in the woods and my twelve-hundred-foot-long driveway has a gate and cameras. My house cannot be seen from the road and nobody just drops by; it's a trek to get here. She knocked on my door and, finding nobody home, walked right in and looked in our refrigerator. I had left the door unlocked, because so many people were checking on our house for us. If we needed someone to bring us something and we couldn't get away, they would be able to do it for us. Since we had been living in Boston for close to a month, I had pitched all the perishable food and milk and there was nothing but a jar of pickles and a bottle of ketchup in the fridge. She went to the grocery store and bought all kinds of food, brought it back, and put it there for us when we returned. She left the note saying to call when I read it.

I couldn't believe it. Of all the people in North America, this Sister of Mercy from my altar boy days, someone whom I hadn't seen or talked to for twenty years, would not have come to my mind as being so insistent to find us and offer help. But there it was. Nobody else went as far as she did to seek us out and take such affirmative action to tend to our needs. She was fearless. In my mind, hers was a quintessential act of Christian charity, and remains a model for all of us to emulate.

We put Molly in the tub, had our supper, and tucked her into her own bed, just like old times. But it was not like old times. Our Katie was gone. That night I sat down at the computer and wrote Katie's obituary. On the way home from Massachusetts, I had called my friend Marion, who owns the funeral home our family has used for generations. She has been a friend of the family for years, as had her father. I never thought I would have to call on her professional services for my child. She had suggested that I write the obituary and email it to her as soon as possible, so she could get it published in the paper in a timely manner. In my naiveté, I included the cause of Katie's death as MRSA pneumonia in the listing. The inclusion of those four letters, MRSA, would prove to be a huge mistake.

The next day, Sunday, started out in a terrible way. I woke up around six in the morning and just lay there in bed, contemplating the enormity of our tragedy. I didn't know what to expect, what might happen, or what to do. We had to take care of Molly, and we had to take care of each other. Cheryl had some leave time from work, and I had not started any big projects, so we could take the time to figure out a plan. I had no idea where to start. I knew I wouldn't be able to work for a while, but I had employees and truck and heavy equipment payments, and thinking about those responsibilities was causing me more stress. Winter was coming, my plow truck wasn't ready, and I had no wood in the wood shed. There was a lot on my mind.

Around seven, I heard Molly wake up and get out of bed. Her little feet hit the floor and she started to come downstairs. But there was no Katie with her. Katie was a light sleeper and every morning, as soon as Molly was up, or sometimes before, Katie would run into her room and squeal with delight to see her sister. Then they would race downstairs together and into our bedroom, where Katie would jump into bed with us and hide under the covers from Molly. Molly would be right on her heels, climbing in any way she could to be part of the show. Not this morning. Molly came down quietly and slowly peeked around the corner from the stairs, and whispered to me, "Daddy, where's Katie?" It was the most painful question ever asked of me.

I helped her up into bed with us and explained that Katie was in heaven now. Molly immediately said, "I know, I saw her, and she looks silly with her angel wings." I asked her what she meant and she told me that when she had seen Katie in the hospital, there were two Katies. There was "one in the hospital bed, and she can't talk right now, and one over the hospital bed, with angel wings." I asked her if Katie had said anything to her, and Molly put her finger to her lips and told me, "She said 'Shh, don't tell Mama you can see me!'"

I was flabbergasted. We had not said anything about angels or angel wings; we tried to be careful about what we said in front of Molly so she would not get upset. Molly was only two-and-a-half years old, yet she claimed to be seeing her sister. It was weird, and there would be more sightings by Molly later.

We debated about going to church that morning, but we agreed that we needed time to ourselves in our own house to absorb things and unwind. I was still in a fog but I wanted to get the funeral business out of the way, so I called the funeral home and made an appointment to meet that afternoon to go over the details.

There are those we meet in life who have certain gifts when it comes to dealing with people. Our funeral director, Marion, is just such a person. Her family has owned the funeral service for several generations, and she and her husband, Charlie, operate it today. Her father was a friend of my parents, and my mother had helped him load many a gurney into the hearse during the thirty-five years she worked at the hospital. He handled the funerals of my maternal grandparents in the 1960s and 1970s, and of my godfather in the 1980s. I knew her father, too, and he was a great guy. I'd known Marion all of my life, but I'd never had to hire her to run a funeral.

When we met at the funeral home, she was pleasant and jovial, but not in a disrespectful or inappropriate way. She sees families at their most distressed and upset times, and guides them through the process with respect and humor in a way that makes them feel better about the grim task at hand. The ringtone on her cell phone plays "When the Saints Go Marching In," which made us laugh.

Cheryl and I would not stand to see a small casket being rolled down the aisle in the church and have it sitting there through the service. We also agreed that we did not want a wake. Because of the postmortem, I knew it would take a lot of work to get Katie present-able for an open casket, and besides, I would not stand to see my little girl laid out in a funeral home. I didn't want to talk to anybody about it. I am sure I could not have made it through the formalities associ-ated with wakes and traditional funerals. We decided to have a private burial in our neighborhood cemetery, with no wake and no casket in the church. Instead, we would ask Father Ray, our parish priest, to come to the cemetery and conduct a committal service and have the Mass for Katie without the casket, after the burial. This would prove to be an important idea.

I have been involved with the cemeteries in my town since I was twelve years old, when my brother and I started mowing the grass with a mechanical reel-type mower and hand clippers. As an adult, I have served as sexton for the cemeteries for decades. The sexton is the person who oversees the cemeteries and keeps track of burials and the placement of monuments and gravestones. In Elizabethan drama, the sexton's job was the lowest class of employment, a job nobody wanted, and as such, offered job security. It is much the same today. In our small town, what records that do exist are poor, and many times one must know several generations of family history and genealogy to locate a gravesite. Even then we sometimes find that people have been buried in a family plot and no one ever recorded it. It is frustrating and embarrassing to have to tell a family that someone is buried in a plot that they thought was open and available for the last thirty years. Funeral directors, the sexton's primary contact, often don't take that kind of news gracefully. One even threatened to call the state police and file a complaint when I couldn't find a gravesite where someone wanted to bury a family member. I had dealt with a lot of different funeral directors during my time as sexton, and none were as easy to deal with as Marion and Charlie. We were glad to have them and left the funeral home feeling secure and relieved. There are few people who could have done that for us at that time, but Marion did. She is a special person, a true professional with a special gift.

In the time of my father, not so long ago, families handled their burials without a sexton. They buried their own, in their family plots. Even today in our town there are some old families who still do it that way. My duties occasionally interjected me into their plans, and I always deferred to the way they wanted to handle it. I waived any town policies that might impact them in a negative way. For example, I let them mark out the grave, dig the hole, and fill it back in without so much as a passing glance at how they were doing it, as long as it was in the right spot. Most of the time, their family records are better than the town's.

In the early 2000s, the patriarch of one of these old families had to bury his son's wife. When he called the town office to tell them when they were going to dig the grave, the administrator told him he had to talk to me before they opened the grave. I had known him for my entire life, so when he called, I asked him how long he had been burying his family members in that cemetery. He thought for a minute and remarked that he had dug his first grave when he was fourteen years old, sometime in the late 1930s. He had been burying family members there for more than sixty years, and since I had been sexton for only twenty-three years, I didn't feel that I had any moral authority to instruct him on what to do. The family took care of their part of the cemetery—to the embarrassment of the town, as their section looked much better than the rest of the cemetery, and had for decades.

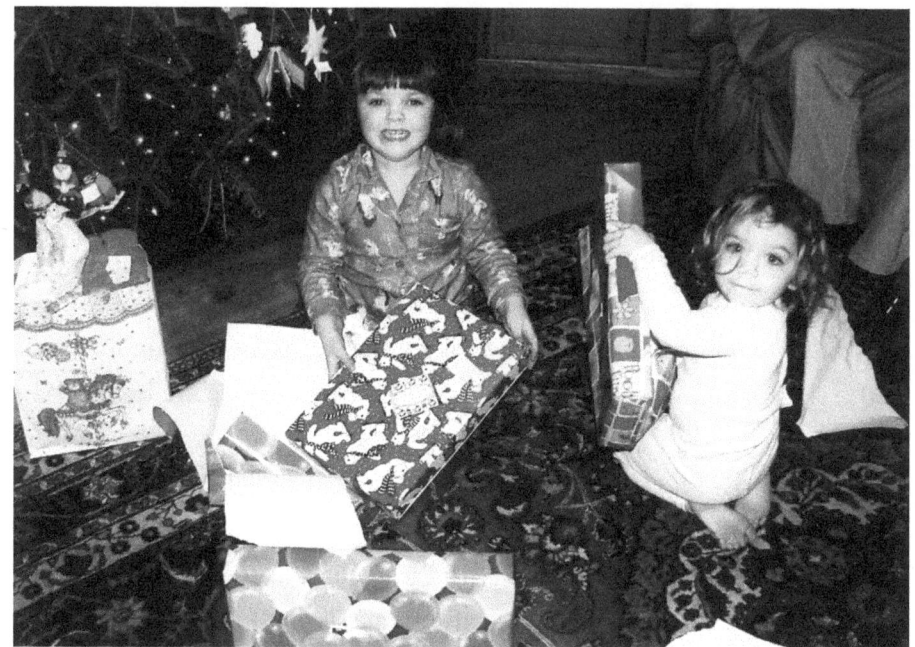

Katie and Molly opening presents.

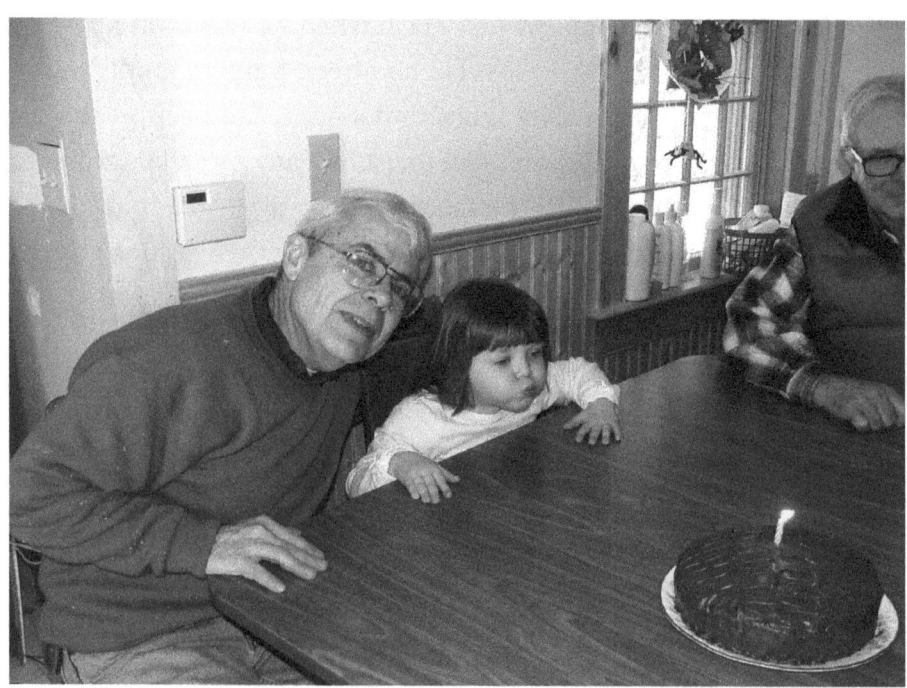

Katie with grandfathers helping to blow out candle on Molly's first birthday.

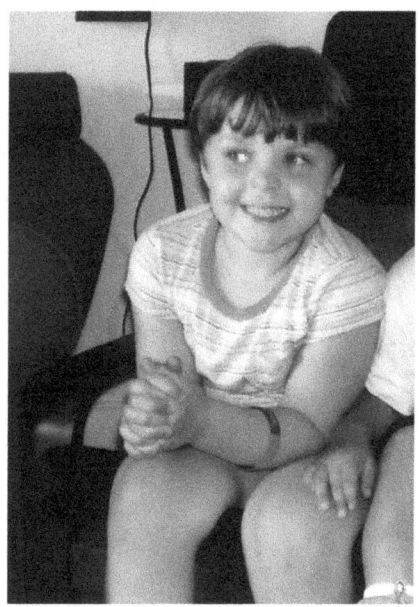

Katie at Auntie Deb's house in South Boston.

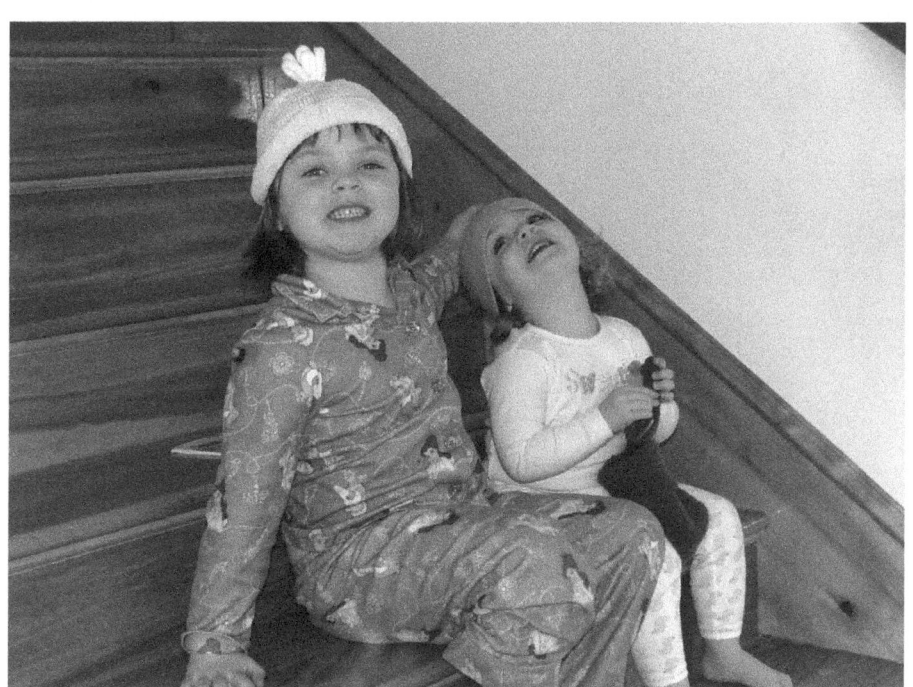

Katie and Molly on the stairs.

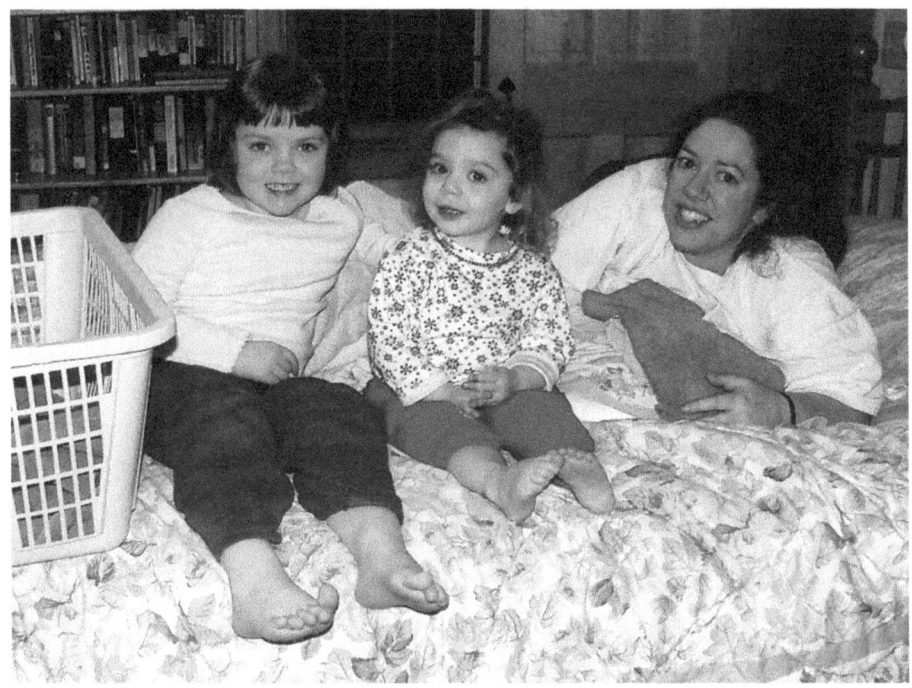

Katie, Molly, and Cheryl folding sheets.

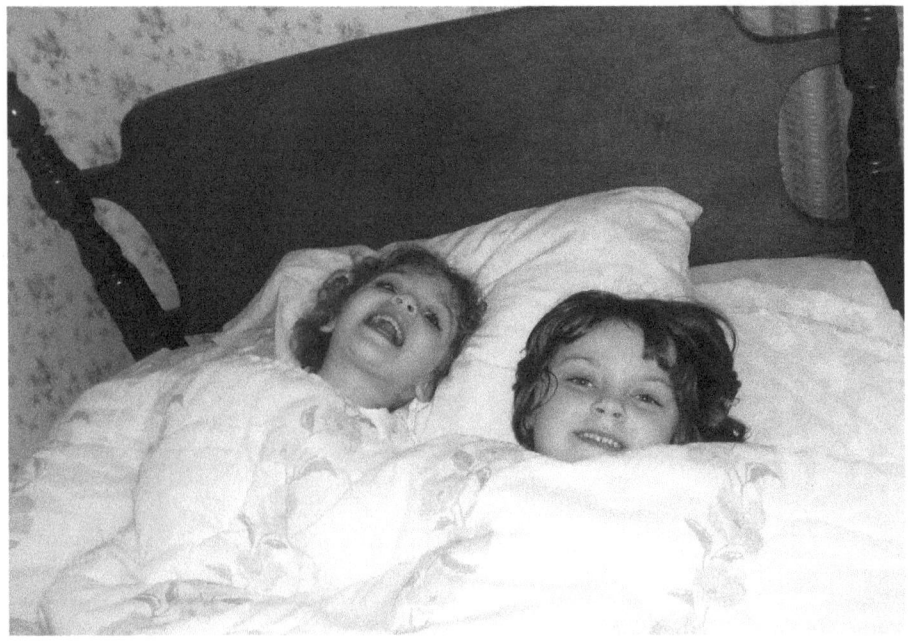

Katie and Molly at grandparents' house getting ready for bed.

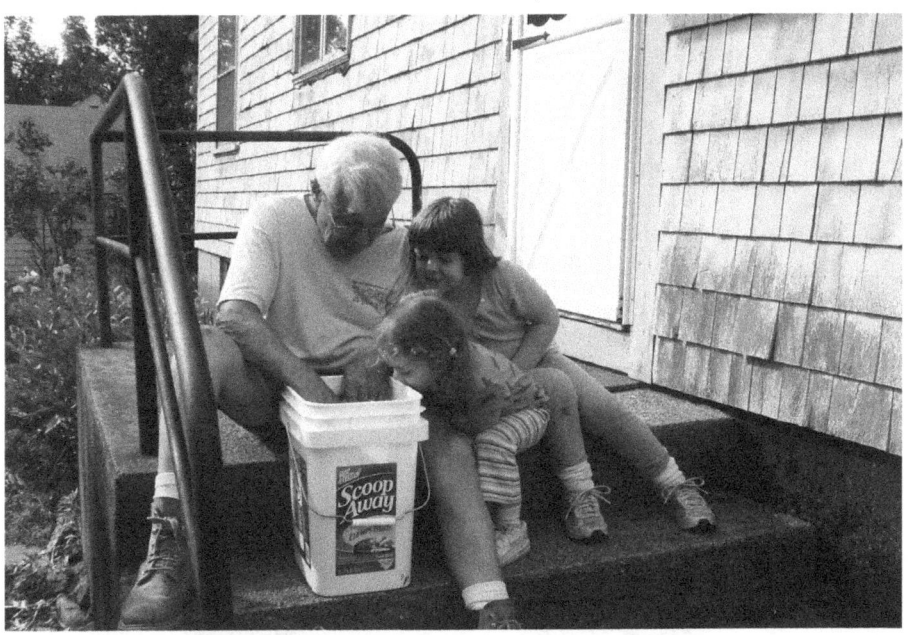

Katie, Molly, and Grandpa Jim sorting blueberries.

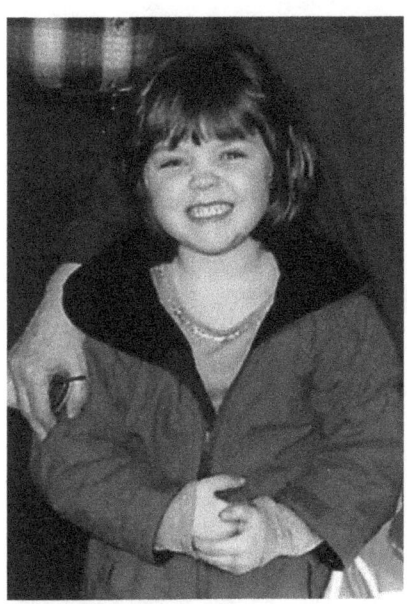

Katie at my parents' house, with my mother's hand on her shoulder.

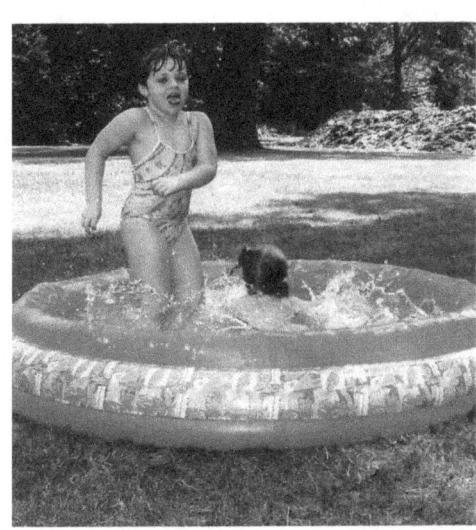

Katie in the kiddie pool at Cheryl's parents' house in North Attleboro.

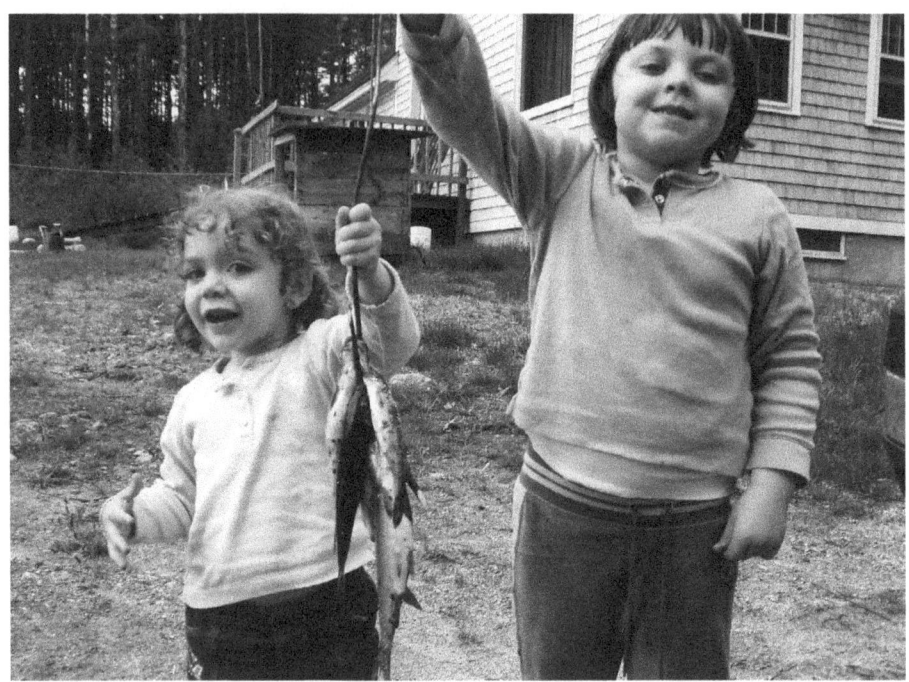

Katie and Molly with fish they caught by themselves.

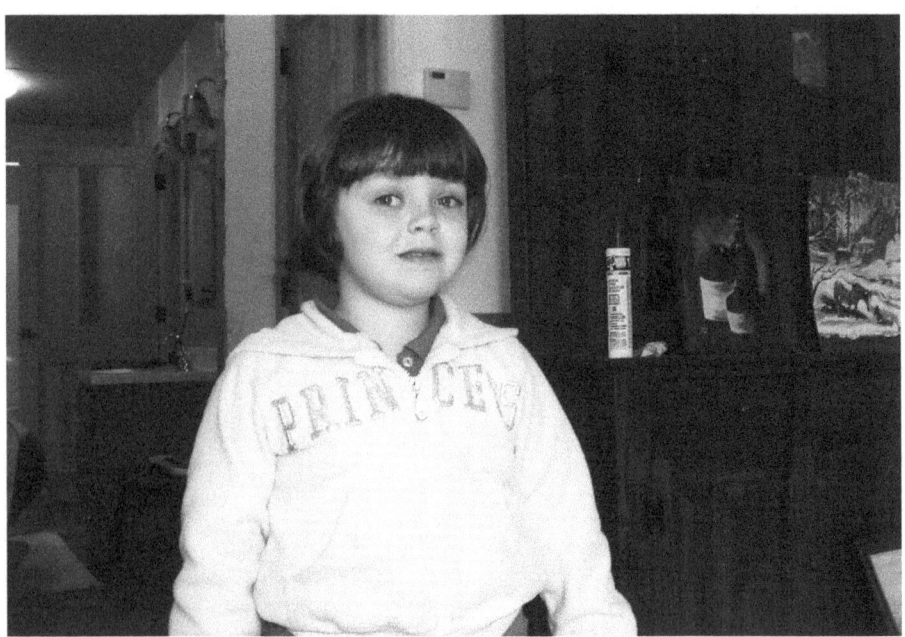

Katie, age four, in our kitchen.

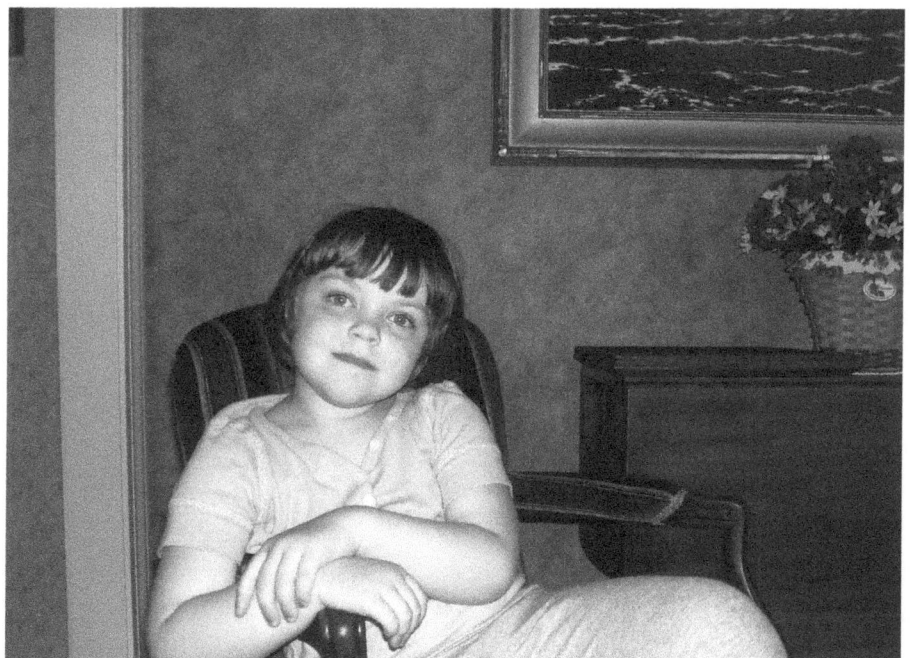

Katie posing in grandparents' living room.

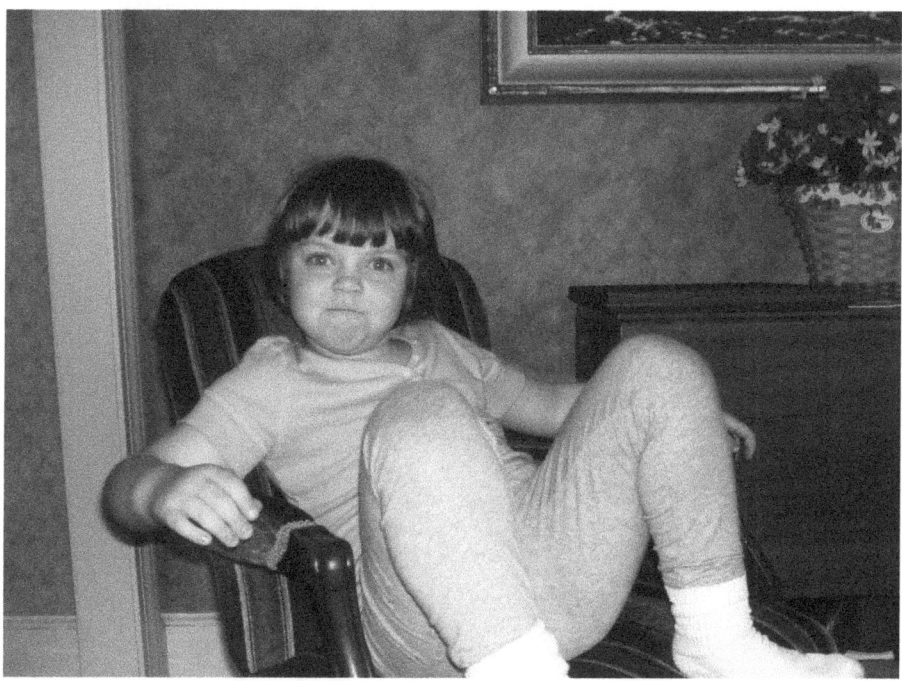

Katie tired of posing in grandparents' living room.

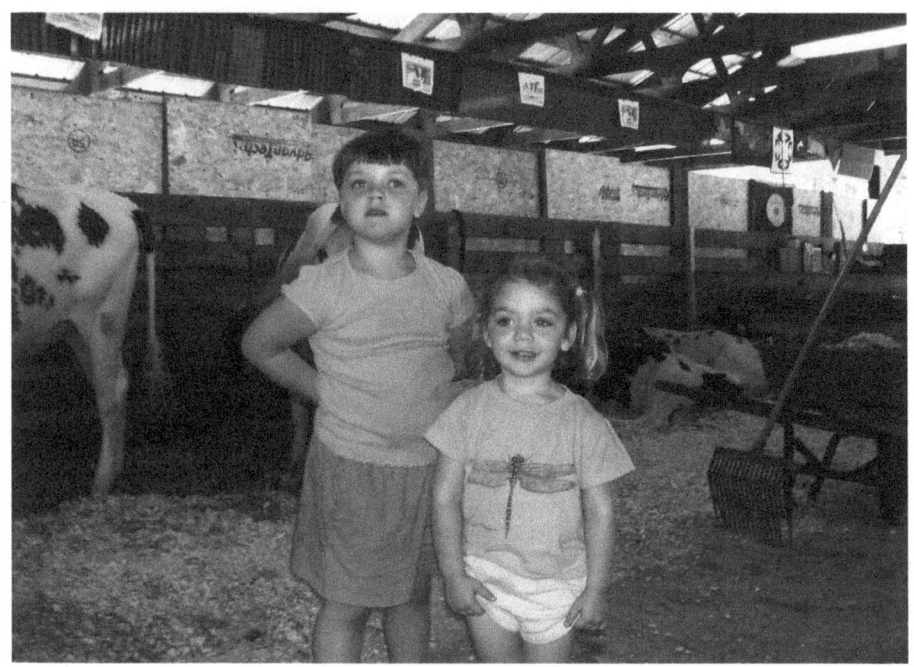

Katie and Molly at the fair with our neighbor's dairy cows.

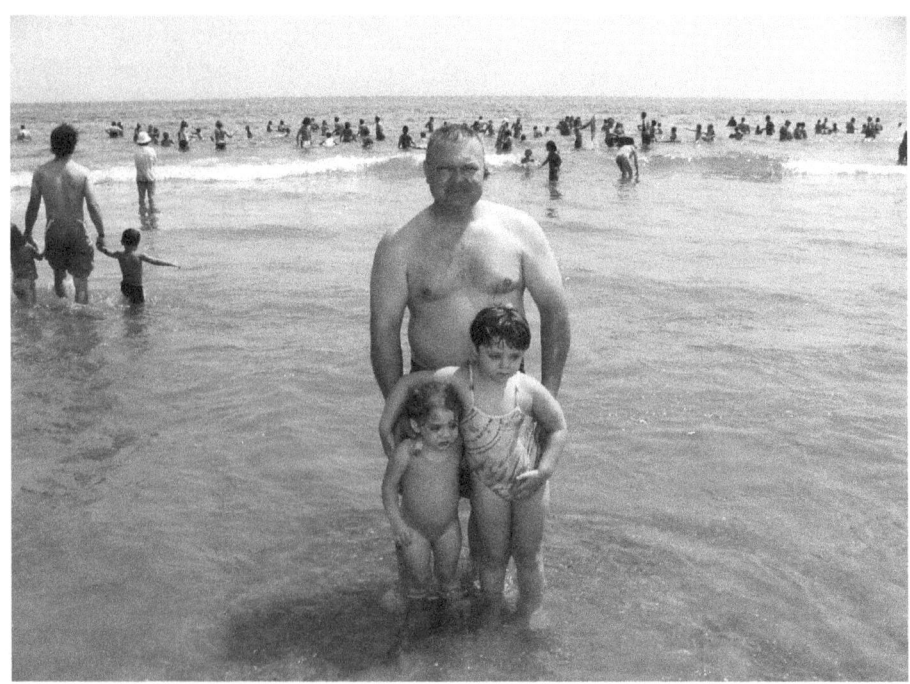

Katie, Molly, and their dad at the ocean.

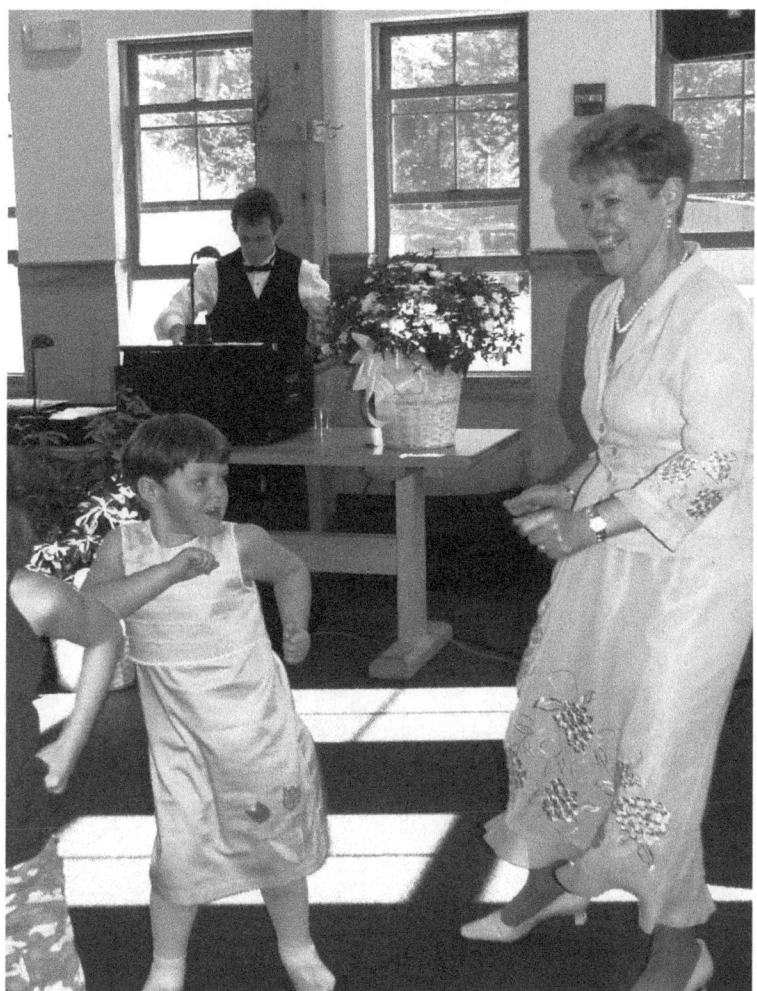

Katie and her grandmother, Ann, at the wedding. Note that Katie has lost her shoes.

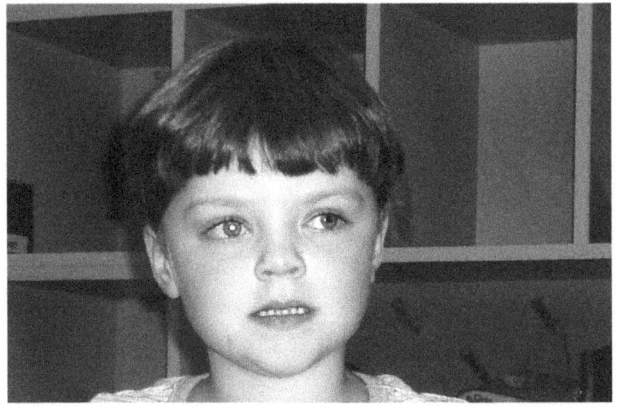

Katie at preschool two weeks before she got sick.

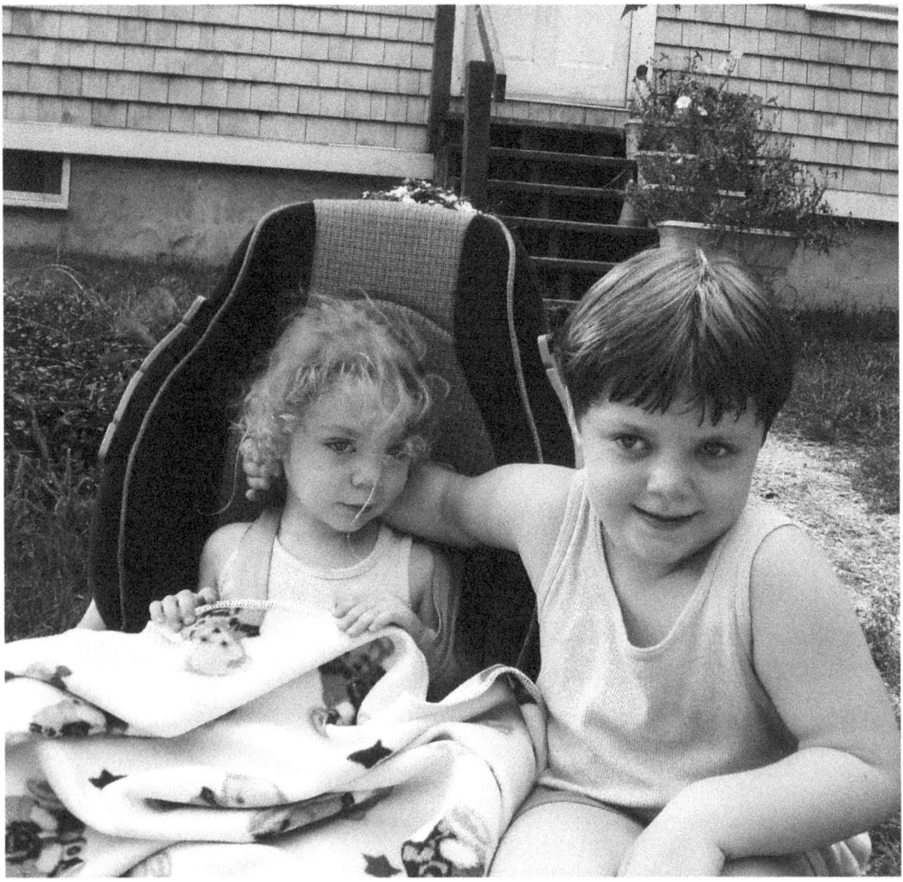

Katie and Molly the day before she got sick. Notice that her eyes look tired.

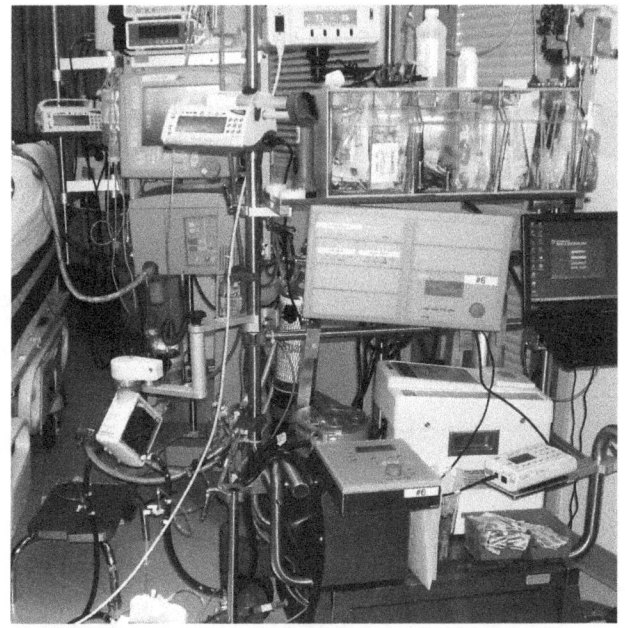

Bedside technology on one side of the bed in Katie's hospital room.

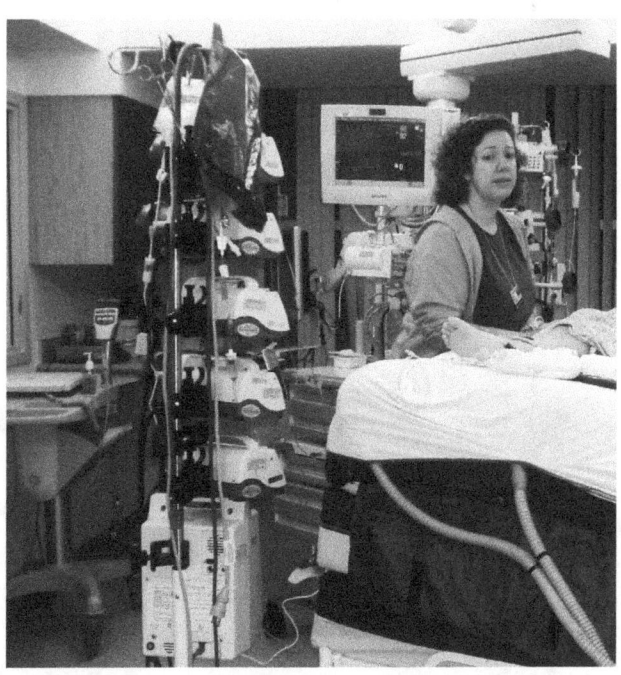

More technology on the other side of the bed. Now on Day 5: notice how tired Cheryl looks.

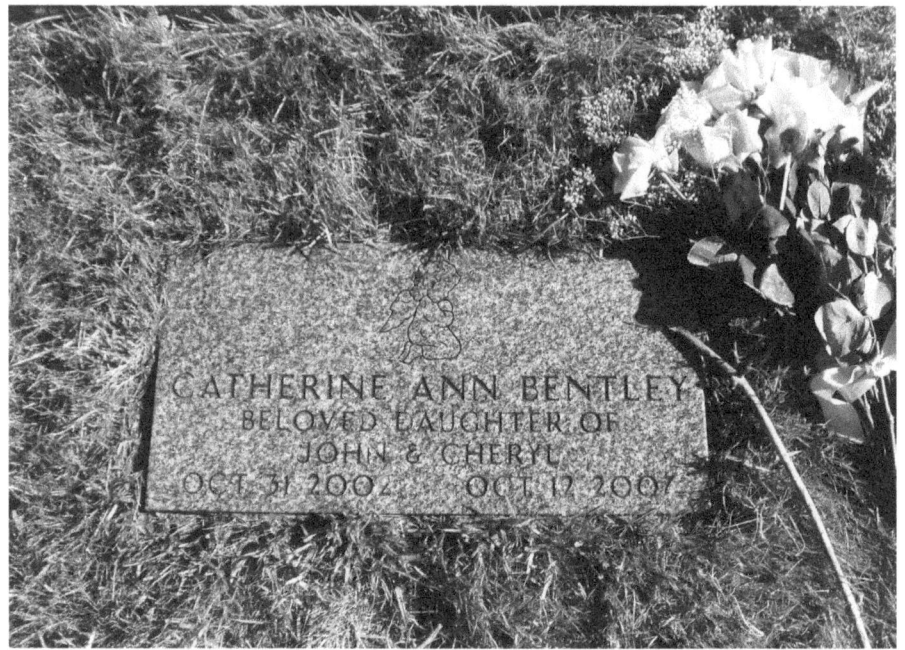

Katie's grave marker at the cemetery.

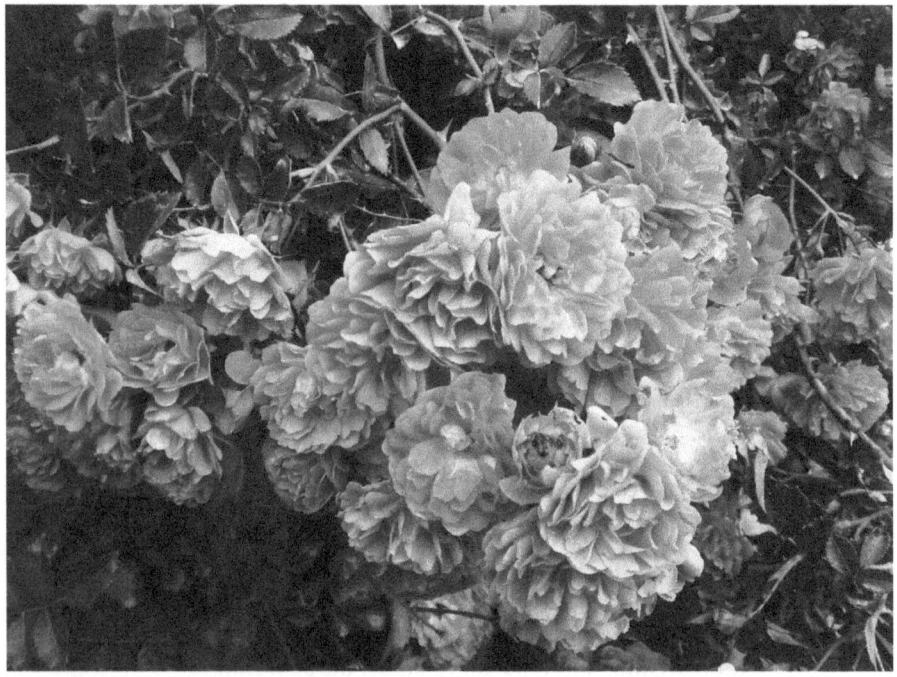

My great-grandmother's rose bush that bloomed so well the next spring.

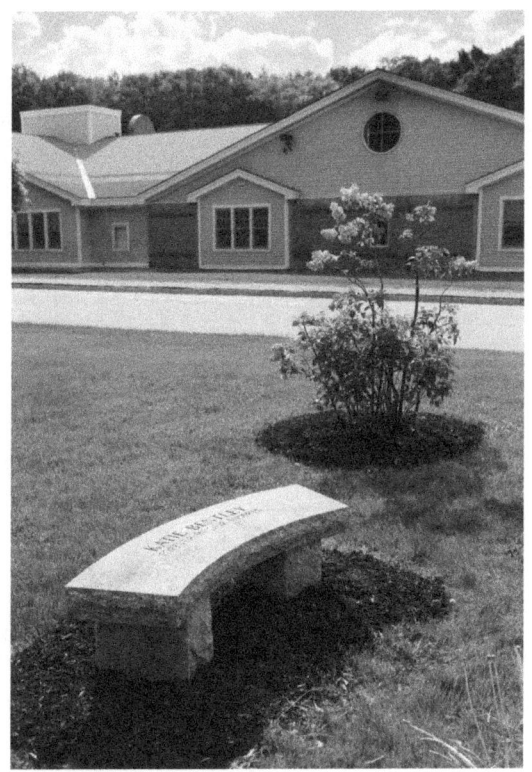

Katie's bench at her preschool.

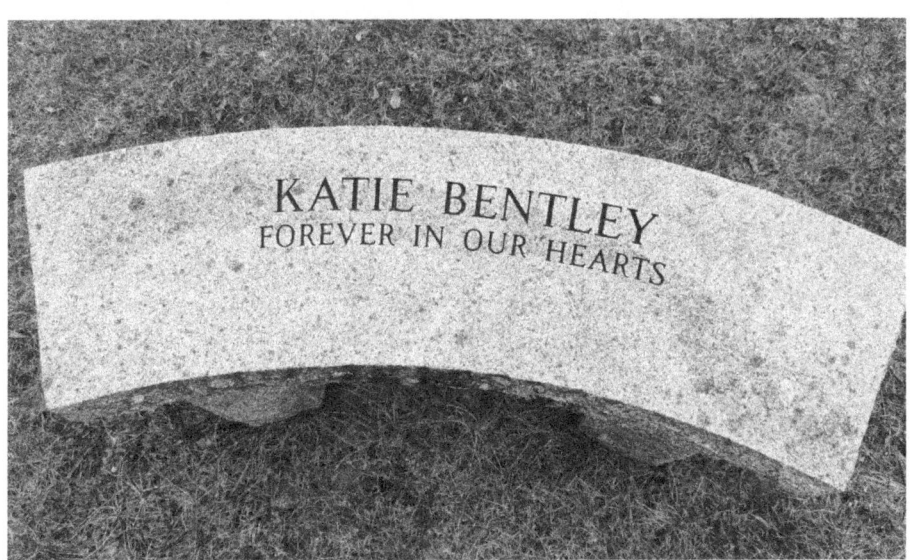

Closeup of Katie's bench.

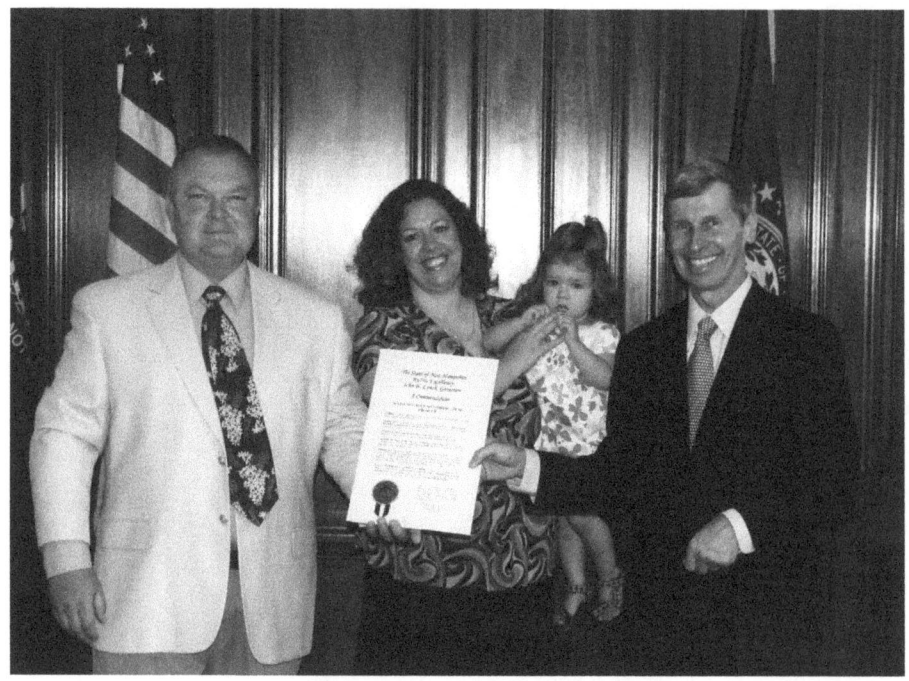

New Hampshire Governor John Lynch presenting us with a proclamation for planting the state flower with the Katie Bentley Lilac Project.

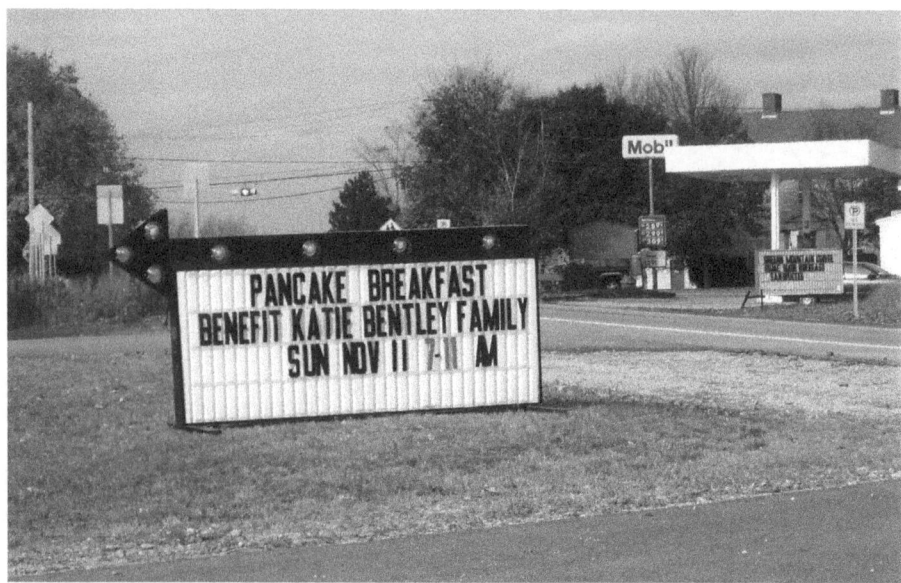

Pancake breakfast sign at the fire station.

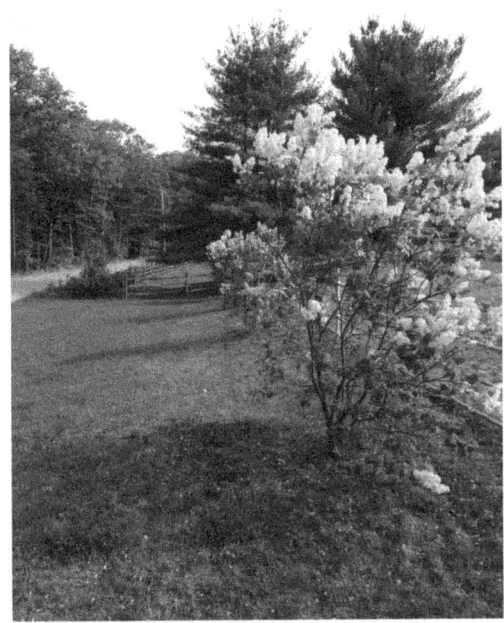

Lilacs at Katie's cemetery.

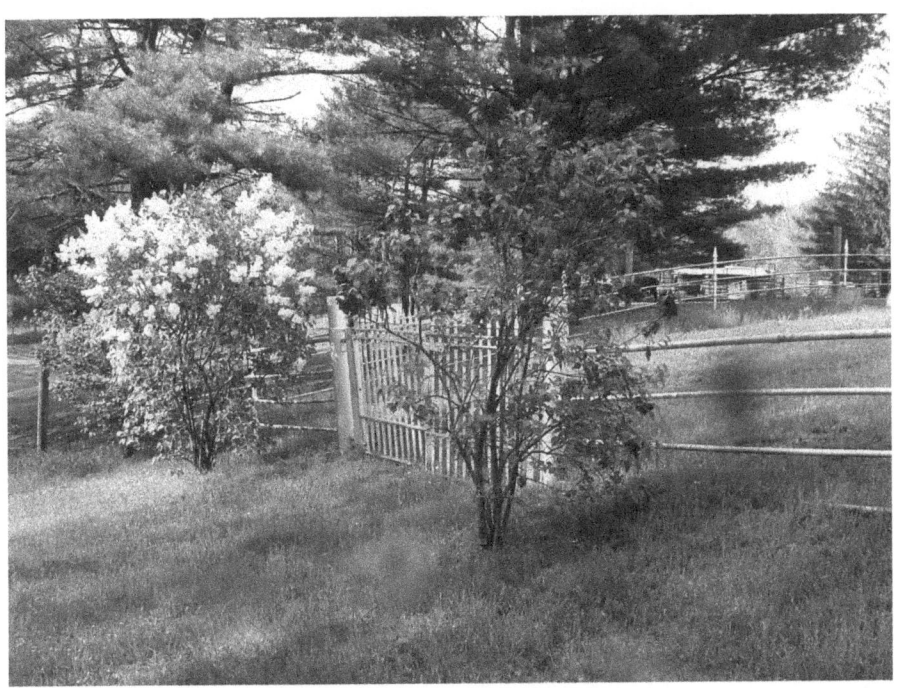

More lilacs at the cemetery.

CHAPTER 9

Storm Clouds with the Press and Visions of Katie

On Monday we had to meet with our priest, Father Ray, to ask him about the funeral arrangements we had outlined with the funeral director. We stopped to visit with my mother on the way. She was uncontrollably upset. We all took Katie's death hard, but my mother was absolutely incapacitated by it. She had been a nurse for forty years and had seen a lot, but I guess it's different with one's own family.

We explained to Father Ray what we wanted, and he was understanding and helpful and tried to cheer us up as best he could. Later I learned that he also was upset by Katie's death. He didn't let it show that day but several months later, he told me that after all his years as a priest, the death of a child was still hard for him to understand. The funeral Mass was set for 10:30 a.m., Saturday, October 20, with a private committal ceremony preceding it at nine at the cemetery. I thought it ironic that Cheryl and I were married on a Saturday at ten thirty so many years ago.

Father Ray offered the use of the parish center gym for a reception and we accepted. We wanted to get it all done and out of the way with the least amount of inconvenience to all involved, including us. We were in no shape for a big production. We needed to get through it alive.

After we left the church, we went to the flower shop and I bought flowers for Cheryl and my mother. As we were leaving the shop, I received a call on my cell phone from the state epidemiologist's staff at the New Hampshire public health office in Concord. Katie's obituary had been published in the newspaper that morning, and the reporters had seized upon the MRSA adjective I had included in it. The caller wanted to alert us that the story was being reported and to warn us we would be receiving a lot of calls. I thanked the person who called and assured her that I had a plan. My plan was to hang up on them. We went to lunch and didn't give it another thought. What followed would prove to be the biggest publicity event that Cheryl and I had ever experienced. None of it was good.

The calls started coming in from newspapers and television stations in New Hampshire that afternoon, and the next day, the national cable stations started covering Katie's death. I talked to one reporter and decided that after that unpleasant interaction, I was not going to take any more calls.

On Tuesday I went to the town office with Molly to buy the cemetery plot for Katie. I know the ladies who work there well. I went to elementary school with their kids, and our families have known each other for several generations. They were upset, but we got the deeds filled out and the transaction done. My parents already owned two lots, so I bought the remaining gravesites beside theirs. Then I headed to the cemetery to mark out the grave.

My uncle and cousin are buried in the lot directly in front of ours. We wanted to keep the family together. When I was born, we lived in a house within sight of the cemetery, and I want to be buried there, where I worked at my first job, mowing the grass. I never thought I would need to bury my child in the same place.

My job as the sexton required me to mark out gravesites, and Molly and Katie would occasionally accompany me when I did the job. They would laugh and run back and forth in the grass while I did my work. Sometimes they would lie on the ground and roll back and forth together, and when the grass was freshly cut, they would get covered in the clippings, laughing all the harder for it. Marking out a grave takes only a few minutes, but they had a ball every time. I marked out the grave and took Molly home.

Cheryl belongs to a quilt guild that meets once a month. That night was their meeting, and she decided to go. Reporters continued to call, but I didn't have the time to talk to them. I avoided them generally, but I knew I would eventually have to talk to some of them. I wanted to encourage them to get the story straight.

While Cheryl was gone to her meeting, Molly and I had fun getting her bath done and eating supper. We played around after we ate and then it was time for stories and bedtime. As I was getting her tucked into bed, Molly told me that Katie was in heaven now. I told her I knew she was in heaven, because that is where little girls go when they die. She said, "No, Daddy, I know Katie is in heaven right now. She told me so tonight. But she still wants Mama. She misses her. She told me so, I saw her all day." One can only imagine how I felt. I didn't know what to say, except that we still love Katie and we miss her, too. Molly went to sleep and I came downstairs in a state of mild shock. I don't believe that a two-year-old could or would make up a tale like this.

Cheryl's parents, Jim and Ann, came for a visit that night, and I told them the story. Jim said he could feel Katie's presence in the house as soon as he walked in the door. Ann couldn't feel it, but Jim insisted he did, and it was very powerful. He did not think it was an emotional reaction. He described it as much the same as what we felt the first time we came home from North Attleboro.

The local paper ran Katie's obituary on Tuesday, along with a story about Katie and the germ that killed her. The article centered on the contagious nature of MRSA, and they interviewed Katie's school principal and the state epidemiologist by phone for commentary.

On Wednesday, a statewide newspaper ran a story about staph infections and mentioned Katie's death. They interviewed an employee of the state public health office for some background information. All she could tell them was to confirm the death of a Concord-area child from MRSA pneumonia. It was easy to figure out who it was, since the obituary had been published the previous day. If I had not put those four letters, M-R-S-A, in the obituary it would have been a guessing game, but those letters identified the decedent.

I called the author of the article and I asked her where she got her information about Katie, because none of our family members had talked to her. I also asked her if she had ever lost a child, and if she had any idea what the family might be going through right now. She agreed to talk to the editors before they ran any more stories. I did not hear back from her again.

When the story broke, the media went wild.

In the age of the internet, stories like this one go worldwide in a matter of hours. The national news media picked it up, and the cable television networks in New York started calling. They called my house four times, which was understandable. But they called my mother and father's house seventeen times in one afternoon. We all have caller ID so we can screen our calls to some degree. I was livid that they would drag my parents into the story to such a degree. My mother was inconsolable, more upset about Katie's death than any other thing that had ever happened in her life. We were concerned that her health might be in jeopardy, that she might have a heart attack or a stroke. To have the reporters badgering her and us was inexcusable. I suppose they feel that they have to "get the scoop," but there are certain boundaries that should not be crossed in pursuit of news. In my mind, this was one of them.

A reporter from a television station called the house, and asked me if I had any comment. I told him my statement was that I thought the reporters were out of control. My only comment was to demand privacy for me and my family, and that no one from his organization or any other should call any of us again. He was polite and offered his apologies for disturbing me and his condolences on our loss. He agreed to not call again. This was a change from my previous interaction with the newspaper reporter, a testament to his greater maturity and experience.

As the story attracted more attention, most of the people who called offered support. My friend the county sheriff called to say he would help us in any way he could. He suggested that we get a spokesman to handle the inquiries. He originally offered to serve as our family spokesman, but the more we talked about it, the more we realized that the mischief makers would negatively exploit the fact that an active-duty law enforcement officer inserted himself into the story. It might make it look like a criminal or investigative case, which it was not. It could also complicate his standing in the event of any civil cases that might arise in the future. He had to stay neutral and out of the spotlight, but he would do whatever he could within those parameters.

I called the New Hampshire governor's office to see if they could help. The governor's press liaison told me he thought it would die down in a few days. In the meantime, he would see what he could do. He called back later that day and told me he had spoken to the other television reporter who was badgering us. This reporter told him that Katie's death was a big story and that the station had to follow the news. The governor's aide insisted that he show some respect for the family. It must have worked, because the reporter did not call us again, though he continued to report erroneous information on TV.

A Boston television station sent a news van to Katie's school and to the town office. They approached the school, the church, anybody and everybody they could think of who might have a comment. It had gone beyond informing the public, and became a feeding frenzy of a particularly non-nutritious kind.

Because of all the coverage, the school began to receive phone calls from parents who were understandably worried about whether what Katie had was contagious. The New Hampshire Public Health Office was right on top of it. The state epidemiologist offered to come to the school and answer questions from parents. A meeting was hastily arranged, and on Wednesday, October 17, the doctor stepped off an airplane returning from an out-of-state conference and drove straight to the school for the meeting. His job is as much about education as it is medicine. Much of what is required of public health officials is to present a calm atmosphere in the face of hysterical reporters who are convinced they have discovered the next plague. I spoke with him in the course of this writing and thanked him for the work he did for us at the time. In his words, his goal is to "right-size" the story, for the reporters and for the public.

One of my attorney friends, Peter, called and offered to help. I asked him if he wanted to serve as the family spokesman, and he readily agreed. I told him that the television reporter had called the church where the funeral was going to be held, and asked them if there were any plans to fumigate the church. He exclaimed, "Oh for the love of God, what is wrong with these people?!" I told him there would likely be TV cameras at the funeral and we needed to be prepared. Peter told me he would talk to the chief of police in Franklin, and I told him about the offer of support from the sheriff. We would have plenty of help to deal with the funeral crowd and interloping reporters.

The frenzy of coverage was starting to get out of hand. Peter agreed to draft a press release and call me back. To my surprise, I received a call from Molly's godmother, Xander. She was now an attorney in Washington, DC, and had been approached at work by her old roommate from law school days. The roommate worked as a "booker" for a national cable news station in DC. This reporter knew Xander was a friend of the family of the little girl who had died, and she wanted to get the story from her, or from us. I told her I had just spoken to Peter, so she said she would contact him concerning a press release. After speaking with the public relations office at her firm, who raised their eyebrows that their newly hired employee would be approached at work by a national cable channel and would need to issue a press release at all, the PR office of a large law firm from Washington, DC, drafted a press release on their letterhead for the national media outlets. Xander sent it to Peter and they agreed to work together on a coordinated approach.

Peter called me back later and told me we could count on the full support of the Franklin Police Department, that the chief would have extra men on duty on Saturday, and that the Merrimack County Sheriff's Department would be there in force as well. That part was beginning to come under control.

Around this time, another old attorney friend called. I had not spoken to him for at least fifteen years, but he had heard about Katie and wanted to know if we needed any help. I had worked with him on political campaigns and I knew him pretty well back then. I had always heard he was an ambulance chaser, but his next statement surprised me. "Do you have the medical records yet?" was his question. I told him I didn't, and I didn't have any plans to get them at the time. He said, "Why don't you get them, and when you do, let's sit down and review them. Maybe I can get you a little money."

There it was—a little money. I was still in a state of shock about Katie's death. I didn't know what to say, so I didn't say anything. I thought about it a lot later on, though, and the more I thought about it, the more I realized how bad things really are in the world today. That day, I thanked him for his concern, then threw his number in the wood stove.

After I had made my phone calls in the morning, I went back to the cemetery to finish digging the grave. My cell phone rang and my brother was on the line. He said he just got home a few minutes ago with his big excavator on the trailer behind the tri-axle dump truck. As he was backing the excavator off the trailer, he looked up to find a Boston news station satellite truck in his driveway. Reporters were milling about, setting up a camera, and they approached him to ask some questions. They saw the last name on his equipment.

They asked if he knew or was related to the little girl who had died, and did he have any comment. As he climbed down out of the excavator, he said that he did have a comment, that they were trespassing, and he challenged them to a race. He told them that if they could beat him to their van, they would win. If he beat them, he was going to use the excavator bucket to crunch up their truck. Then they would have a real story. They literally ran back to their van, quite sure they were out of their element way up in the woods of New Hampshire.

I told him I was working on the grave and he could just come along when he was ready. He was bringing the mini excavator to finish digging the hole. As soon as we hung up, the phone rang again. The same news crew was now at the town office, which was closed, but the town administrator was there and went out to see what they wanted. She offered no comment and sent them on their way, but she called me to warn me that they were afoot.

I had worked on the county sheriff's campaigns for office for years. He always told me if I ever needed help, he would be there. I decided now was the time to ask him for help, and I called him. He asked me where everybody was. I told him I was trying to dig the grave and I did not want the cameras recording me doing it, and the news van was roaming all over town seeking interviews. He rolled out the cavalry, sending cruisers to the town office, to my brother's house, and to my place. I had to go back to the house for more tarps and when I got there, our town police chief was in the driveway with my father. They were looking for trouble, but luckily, no reporters had yet arrived. Dad agreed to stay at my house until I was finished and the chief was going to go look for the news van. It was totally ridiculous.

My cousins started calling. My older cousin, Tim, had heard about the trouble with the reporters and was on his way over right then. He lived a few towns away and it would be a few minutes before he arrived. He agreed to physically remove any reporters who showed up at either my parents' house or mine. Cousin Tim is a huge man, more than six feet tall, strong and fearless, with a long black beard and black ponytail. He usually wears biker leather, but even without it, when he is angry—and he was—he looks like a dangerous man. He agreed to serve as one of the family bodyguards on Saturday at the burial and funeral, and was ready to be arrested if necessary. His younger brother, Tom, who shared my father's birthday, March 26, is also a big man and was recently honorably discharged from the US Army after several tours in the Middle East as a helicopter mechanic. These two brothers were ready for anything that came up, including getting arrested. It was reassuring to know we could count on them when the chips were down. My brother and I finished digging the grave and I went home to relax.

At six o'clock that evening, all the major networks ran stories on Katie's death. Her picture from the obituary was on TV for several days afterward. Friends of mine whom I hadn't talked to for twenty years or more were calling, all offering to help. I simply could not talk to everyone. I was in no state to talk anyway, my voicemail was full, and I couldn't do any more. I was overwhelmed. The barrage of inquiries from all types of journalists was unprecedented in either my or Cheryl's experience. It seemed to feed on itself; we had never seen anything like it. We both had given interviews or commentary to public media outlets, but they were usually about mundane political issues or for the various nonprofit groups to which we belonged. We withstood it thanks to our many friends in public office who stepped up to help. We had deputy sheriffs parked at the end of my driveway and my brother's and parents' driveways, and at the school and the town office. They seemed to be everywhere at once. New Hampshire Governor John Lynch's office talked to the reporters and urged them to show restraint and respect.

It was never clear what they wanted. They hyped up the MRSA component of the story, but never checked, or if they did, never reported about how rare it was. It was an irrational pursuit, and the invasion of our privacy was not a concern for them. Our phones rang nonstop, and eventually we just had to unplug them. We needed time to absorb the loss, and peace and quiet to heal. We didn't get it until much later.

The next day, Thursday, I bought some *NO PARKING* signs for the cemetery. It's located on a narrow country dirt road with limited visibility on the approach. We didn't know how many people might show up, but it would not be good to have too many cars parking and blocking the narrow road. We wanted a private burial, but that could be in jeopardy now. We treated the time and location of the service like top-secret information, telling only a few close friends and our family members about it. The last thing we needed was a gaggle of reporters badgering grieving family members, with our escape route blocked by parked cars. When I stopped at my parents' house, I noticed there were no flowers on my mother's kitchen table, so I went to the flower shop and bought another nice arrangement for her. I wanted to cheer her up in any way I could.

I arrived home and my attorney Peter called to say he had the press release ready. After getting my approval, he released it to the New Hampshire media outlets on his letterhead, rather than on that of the big Washington, DC, law firm. He thought we should wait before releasing it to the national news networks, lest it incite them to more "investigative" reporting.

For Immediate Release

From: Attorney Peter Fitzpatrick on behalf of the Catherine Bentley family.

Statement of the Bentley Family Regarding the Death of Catherine Bentley

The Bentley family would like to express its deep sadness over the loss of Catherine Bentley and would like to reiterate its desire for privacy and solitude during this time of mourning. It respectfully requests that in doing their jobs the media recognize the solemnity of the situation and respect the family's desire to grieve in private.

The family would also like to take the opportunity to express its sincere gratitude to the doctors and nurses at the hospital in Boston for their heartfelt efforts to care for Catherine.

The family will not be entertaining media requests at this time. Any further inquiries should be directed to the family's attorney, Peter Fitzpatrick.

It worked. The reporters stopped calling us, but I never asked Peter if anybody called him. We had too much going on, and I knew he could handle it.

On Friday, we met with Charlie, the funeral director. He had the brochures ready for the funeral, so we met him at a pizza restaurant that was exactly halfway between our house and the funeral home. At that time, it was managed by my other cousins, and I knew we could count on some privacy. They would eagerly throw out any reporters or other people who might bother us.

The brochures were attractively done and had Katie's picture on the inside cover. The front cover was a picture of a country road in the fall with beautiful foliage, and later, people thought it was our driveway. In reality it was from a collection of standard brochure pictures the funeral home had on file. I wrote the story about Katie that was on the inside and sent it via email, so they could get it printed fast. The text can be found in the appendix.

After we got home, I went over to the church to help set up the tables and chairs for the reception in the gym, but when I got there, it was all done. Church volunteers and the Knights of Columbus had pitched in and finished the job for us. They were putting the finishing touches on the tablecloths and everything looked in order. My friend and neighbor, Melanie, who lived in our old house near the cemetery, was serving as the food coordinator, and the church people and she had called a number of people who volunteered to cook. There are no caterers around this part of New Hampshire.

I left the church and went to the photo lab to pick up pictures of Katie that Cheryl had ordered to assemble into a collage for the reception. Her parents were coming that night and she and her mother were going to make some sandwiches and make the collage. They arrived at six, and her sister Debbie and Tim at nine. That night, when Cheryl and her mother were making the collage, I was drawn to one of the pictures she picked out to use. It was of Katie and me sitting on a bench at a state park on the New Hampshire seacoast.

We always try to get to the ocean at least once in the summer. The water is usually too cold to swim, but the girls like to splash and play and look for seashells. Just two months before Katie got sick, we went for the day to Wallis Sands in Rye. It was hot that day, the first time in years that I remember the water being warm enough to swim in, and swim we did. We took a break to eat lunch, and Katie and I sat on a bench to eat our sandwiches. Cheryl took a picture of us sitting on the bench and we filed it away. That night I noticed there was a plaque on the back of the bench, visible between us where we were sitting. I was intrigued. I enlarged it on the computer and the plaque read, *Donated by Compassionate Friends, Seacoast NH Chapter*. I was dumbfounded. Here we were, two months before she died, sitting on a bench donated by an organization dedicated to helping parents who have lost a child. I took it as a message, but I didn't know what it might mean.

We made two hundred sandwiches for the reception and Cheryl and Ann made the collage of pictures. Things were falling into place on time. Now we had to get through the hard part.

CHAPTER 10

The Funeral

Saturday, October 20, dawned bright and clear, a classic fall morning with stunning foliage for a backdrop. It smelled like fall. We wanted a small, private burial for our Katie girl. We did not put it in the published obituary for that reason. The family and few close friends we had invited started to arrive at our house about eight. We convoyed to the cemetery and arrived a few minutes before nine to find the casket on the grave and covered with flowers. There were a few people already there, including Father Ray, and thankfully, no reporters. The chief of police was there with the cruiser, but he didn't have to intercept any mischief makers. My cousins were there looking big and strong and sharp in their suits, with fire in their eyes, watching for any trouble.

I have buried a lot of people in my town and other town cemeteries over the years. It's the little caskets that are the hardest to do, even though I might not know the families well. This one was nearly unbearable for me. I'm sure it was the same for the others assembled there. The casket looked outstanding. We chose it from a picture in a catalog, but here in real life, it looked mighty fine. Brilliant, shining white and covered with flowers, it was a fitting vessel for my little girl.

Those gathered with us were subdued. Often at funerals, especially Irish funerals like we have on my mother's and wife's sides of the family, there are pockets of joviality and laughter, as people remember the humorous side of the deceased. Not today. There was no laughter, only sadness—deep, profound, ineffable sadness. Those who spoke to me, my closest family members and friends, did not know what to say. What could they say? The little gleaming casket covered with flowers said it for them. Most of my aunts and uncles and cousins were there, some of whom I had not seen for years.

Outside of our nuclear family, Katie's death seemed to hit my father's older brother, Kerry, the hardest. He served in the Korean War in the special forces as a forward observer for field artillery behind enemy lines, a job not known for its high survival rate. He had seen and lived with death up close and imminent over there. He later served as the personal bodyguard to five-star general Mark Clark. In civilian life he was a high-voltage utility lineman, who worked inches away from death every day. He buried a lot of friends over the years who got too close to the wires, and had buried his wife a few years earlier. He and I were close and he loved Katie and Molly. He was tough, tougher and braver than most people, but I could tell it rattled him to the core. He was a wreck.

There were a few chairs set up next to the grave, intended for me and Cheryl, but we insisted that my mother and father and uncle take them. This was the part we had been dreading. This was the end, the final act. The church service would be just an epilogue. In the church one enjoys the comfort of the familiar, the comfort of counsel and fellowship, the acknowledgement and support of civilization and evidence that life does go on. Not here, not now. My Katie girl was in that casket and that casket was going in the ground, and the dirt would go in on top. I had done it many times before and I knew exactly what came next. It was awful. I stiffened my spine and set my jaw, and leaned into the job at hand.

Cheryl did well through it all. Molly kept tugging at her arm, asking what we were doing, what was going on. Molly asked me who was in the casket and I told her it was Katie. She told me that it couldn't be Katie, because she knew Katie was in heaven. It was hard to explain to a little girl of two and a half. My mother did not do so well. She was devastated. Katie was closest to her after me and Cheryl, and Katie's death was an unbearable burden for her. She made it through the service,

God only knows how. My father, a son of the Silent Generation and the Great Depression, never said a word. There was nothing to say.

Father Ray invited us all around the casket, started the service with a few statements, and the curtain opened on the final act. He began the Roman Catholic committal rite:

> *"In the name of the Father, the Son, and the Holy Spirit, Amen.*
>
> *"The life which Catherine received from her parents is not destroyed by death. God has taken her into eternal life. As we commend Katie to God and commit her body to the earth, let us express our common faith in the Resurrection. As Jesus was raised from the dead, we, too, are called to follow Him through death to the glory where God will be all in all . . ."*

Sprinkling the casket with holy water, he said:

> *"We sprinkle Katie's body with Holy Water that recalls her baptism. Since the day she was baptized, she has been entitled to call God her Father and to look forward to spending eternity with Him in heaven."*

And then, together with us:

> *"Our Father, who art in Heaven, hallowed be Thy name, Thy kingdom come, Thy will be done, on earth as it is in heaven. Give us this day our daily bread, and forgive us our trespasses, as we forgive those who trespass against us, and lead us not into temptation, but deliver us from evil. Amen.*
>
> *"Let us pray:*
>
> *". . . May her soul and the souls of all the faithful departed, through the mercy of God, rest in peace. Amen."*

It was over in a few minutes: simple, direct, and traditional. There was silence during the service, and afterward. Nobody looked up; they just looked away and started to leave the graveside, not sure about what to do next. Should they come over and talk to us, or wait, or head to Franklin for the Mass? People milled about, murmuring to each other and casting furtive glances at us. Father Ray answered the question that no one dared ask. He invited us to the church in Franklin for the Mass and a reception immediately following. That was it. It was over. Twenty minutes, and done. Since time was short, we couldn't stay long; we had to get over to the church for the service. Who knew what kind of circus awaited us? We were not looking forward to it.

My brother had helped me with some gravesites over the years. He and his friend, Mike, agreed to stay and fill in the grave after the casket was lowered into the vault. It meant that he would miss some of the service, but it was an important job and he wanted to do it, for us and for Katie. We left and let him tend to the grim task of burying his niece. I had originally planned to do it, but the church service couldn't be pushed out any further than ten thirty, so I would not have time to do both. My brother and my mother talked me out of helping to fill in the grave anyway.

When we arrived at the church there were police cruisers with flashing lights everywhere. There were two deputy sheriffs in uniform in the street directing traffic in front of the church, stopping each car and asking if the occupants were members of the family. This was their way of discovering if any reporters were present. There were several uniformed officers stationed at the front doors of the church. As we pulled in, I counted four cruisers on the street with lights flashing, two from the Franklin Police Department and two from the sheriff's department.

There was a spot reserved for us in the front row of the parking lot. After we parked and started walking toward the front door, I could see two more cruisers tucked in off the street, just up from the church. There were several men in uniform at the entrance to the church and two or three more in the foyer on the inside. The church has three entrances and there were at least two uniformed officers at the two side doors we could see. Inside the foyer stood my two burly cousins in suits, watching intently as each person came in. As we walked down the aisle to the reserved seats in the front row, I recognized more officers in street clothes sitting among the congregation, including in the pews directly behind where we were to be seated. I'm sure there were more whom I didn't see, but it was clear they were ready for trouble, should trouble find its way there.

I saw my attorney Peter sitting there, and Dr. Connor, Katie's doctor. I wanted to invite him to sit with us up front, but I was afraid that he might be recognized as someone other than an ordinary civilian should the cameras arrive. I wanted to spare him the gauntlet and let him remain anonymous. I saw Katie's dentist, but I couldn't take the time to thank any of them just now. We had to get through it.

Later I learned that the Franklin Police Department had five officers on duty that morning, with two assigned to cover the funeral, and there were several sheriff's deputies assigned there, too. The lieutenant in charge of the department told me they had put all of the off-duty officers, including the chief, on standby. Several years later I found out there were sixteen officers stationed in and around the church. I also learned that the surrounding towns had been alerted and had officers on standby should there be a real problem with traffic or crowd control, or with me and my brother and cousins beating up the cameramen. The parking lots were full and people were parking on the street blocks away on both sides of the roads.

Molly's godmother, Xander, and her husband convoyed to the church with us and sat behind us in the second row. Our friends Sande and Tina sat with us and gave all their attention to Molly, trying to keep her quiet. The church was mobbed. I had never seen so many people there, not even during Christmas or Easter Mass. Father Ray estimated there were more than five hundred people, since every seat was full and there were people standing in the entryways, even outside. It was staggering and humbling to me and Cheryl to have so many of our friends and neighbors come to pay their respects.

Father Ray asked me if I had anybody to do the readings for the Mass. I didn't. I asked Xander, and my friend and former lawyer, Liam, if they would do it. Liam is a colorful lawyer, having run for governor once, and I knew he could speak well in public. Xander was great, the best speaker there. She was poised and steady, spoke well, never missed a beat. Their example gave all of us strength and fortitude.

Katie's teachers all sat together and wore ribbons of Katie's favorite color, purple, in her memory. The school nurse read a short eulogy that made everybody cry. She got through it, but told me later she had to practice it for three days to say it without crying. She said:

> *"We at the Boscawen Elementary preschool were truly blessed to know and love you, Katie. You were a part of our family for the last two years and a bright light in our day. Your energy and zest for life put smiles on our faces and laughter in our hearts. You always offered wonderful hugs and were very caring to your teachers and friends.*
>
> *You helped us to appreciate the power of the word 'No.' Even a four-year-old understands what they want to do. This presented us with the challenge of thoughtful manipulation. Because of you, Katie, we are much more creative with all of your friends when they say 'No.' You reminded us that no matter how difficult the 'grown-up' world can be, the simplest things—like a hug, 'I love you,' or sharing your Play-Doh—are what is really important. If the halls at school were ever too quiet, we put you on the purple tricycle. Your laughter echoed down the halls, and even the big kids wanted to ride. You had an amazing understanding of fear in others, and offered your hand to walk your friends to the nurse, visit the Queen in the office, or be the leader in the hall during leprechaun hunts or reindeer leaping. 'See,' we would say, 'do it like Katie. She is having fun, she isn't scared, and she is taking turns.' Katie, you could teach the others to share, and be a best friend to all. That would make our job way too easy!*
>
> *Katie, you will always hold a special place in our hearts. Your friends were blessed to have you in their lives. We only hope we can begin to share your love, enthusiasm, and spirit for life every day in preschool. There will always be purple paintings hanging on the walls of your classroom as the simplest reminder of your presence with us. We love you, and we will miss you terribly."*

I was in a daze, partly from the shock and partly from sleep deprivation. There was a lot going on around me of which I was not particularly aware. Some of our friends sat on the end of our pew, and the plan was for them to occupy Molly if she became rambunctious. I was vaguely aware of Sande and Tina tending to Molly at the other end of the bench.

When Father Ray addressed the congregation, he spoke to us as what I call a ground-level guy, as though he were talking to each of us as individuals and informally. The first thing he said as he took the pulpit was, "Well, this just doesn't make any sense. Death is stupid." I think we were all surprised to hear a priest say that.

The Roman Catholic church believes that baptized children who die before attaining the age of reason, seven years of age, are incapable of committing a sin and therefore are assured salvation. He reminded us of that part of church teaching during the homily. I thought about how much trouble we had endured getting Katie, and then Molly, baptized. When Katie was born, we were going to have her baptized at the church I had attended as a child and young adult and where I had served as an altar boy, though we had been going to a different church that was much closer for years. The priest at that church was a good friend of mine. Two weeks before Katie's scheduled baptism, the priest committed suicide. Rumors swirled about it but we never really knew the reason. I knew him well, he was a good friend, a real intellectual, and it troubled me beyond the inconvenience of having to baptize Katie elsewhere.

Because of the timing, we had gone to Massachusetts to have her baptized by the Irish-American priest who married us, so naturally, when Molly came, he wanted to baptize her, too. Two weeks before Molly's scheduled baptism, he took a leave of absence from the parish. We were left hanging again. We had been attending Mass in Franklin for a while so it made perfect sense to have Molly baptized there. Father Ray was happy to do it, and finally we had two Christian children.

After he delivered his homily, he continued the Mass with the Prayer of the Faithful for Katie:

"Lord God, you entrusted Katie to our care and now you embrace her in your love. Take Katie in your keeping, together with all the other children who have died. Comfort us, your sorrowing servants, who seek to do your will and to know your saving peace. We ask this through Christ, our Lord. Amen."

The mass continued in its regular format until, at last, it was over. We never sit up front when we go to church, but today we had reserved seating. This allowed us to be the first ones out, right behind Father Ray. I wanted to get as far away as I could as fast as I could. We didn't want to form a receiving line in the entrance, but we were partly trapped. We found our escape when Dr. Connor came through. We excused ourselves and walked him to his car in the parking lot across the street.

After the service we had a reception in the gymnasium on the church grounds, part of the old Catholic school that was in session for years but was now closed. My father had attended school there in the 1940s. There were far more people than we had expected. We ran out of food. There's usually a reception line at such events, where every person there comes by and shakes your hand and tells you how sorry they are for your loss. We couldn't bear to do it. With five hundred people it would have taken all day. We stayed for an hour and then decided we had to go home. It was done, and we were still alive. Now, perhaps, the healing could begin.

CHAPTER 11

The Start of Recovery and Seeking the New Normal

On the Tuesday after the funeral, October 23, the television and radio stations were still running an occasional story about Katie, but the phone calls had stopped. At nine in the morning, the house phone rang. I answered to find the governor of New Hampshire, John Lynch, on the phone, calling to check on our welfare, offer his support, and ask if there was anything he could do for us. I was surprised. I'd never had a governor call me at home before that day. Any conversations I had had in the past with a governor had always been business or politics related. I didn't know what to say. He told me his people were talking to the reporters and encouraging them to leave us alone. He closed the call by giving me his personal cell phone number and told me to call him if there was anything else he could do. It speaks to the quality of human being he is, quality that sets politics aside for the service of people. John Lynch is a solid man and a true public servant.

The amount of effort and support directed toward us was enormous. We remain humbled by the sheer number of people, especially in government, who stepped up to do what they could. Because her death was such a big news story and carried as the lead item in local, state, and national television, newspaper, and radio for weeks, everybody knew about it and was talking about it. The invasion of privacy we suffered at the hands of the media was disgraceful. During the years when I was involved in politics, I met a lot of prominent people, many of whom became my friends. Political disputes sometimes result in lawsuits, so I met a lot of lawyers and judges, and I never lost a case. It helps to explain why so many people in government got involved. The rest of the support we received was simply the reaction of our fellow humans, who recognized the enormity of our loss and wanted to do anything they could.

The week after the funeral, on Thursday, October 25, the paper ran an article titled "An Autumn Miracle," about some purple lilacs that were in bloom beside Interstate 89 in Concord. Lilacs bloom in the spring. To have them flower at this time of year was unheard of in New Hampshire. The nurse at Katie's preschool, knowing that purple was Katie's favorite color, cut out the article and mailed it to us, convinced it was a sign from Katie. It was a sign, to be sure, and I missed it. I filed the article and her note away and forgot about it.

One day, sometime in late October, Molly came downstairs in the morning. I was already up and eating breakfast, but Cheryl was still sleeping. Without preamble, Molly told me that Katie was in heaven, that she liked it there and she was playing with a little girl. She said Mary was watching them and they were okay. I told her I was sure Katie was in heaven and that she could see Mary. "No, Daddy, you don't understand. Not little Mary, but big Mary, like in the hospital room." By little Mary, she was referring to a small plastic statue of the Virgin Mary that my mother had given to Katie years ago. Katie took the statue with her everywhere. She even snuck it into daycare on occasion and I would find it in her cubicle when I picked her up in the afternoon. She took it to bed every night and had to have it with her all the time. It was more than just a toy to her.

I asked Molly what she meant about Mary in the hospital room. She said, "When I saw Katie in the hospital room, Mary was in the room, too, when Katie couldn't talk. That's the Mary who is watching Katie and Elizabeth." I asked her who Elizabeth was, and she told me she was the little girl with whom Katie was playing in heaven. I didn't know what to say or how to respond, except to say that I knew Katie was in heaven and we were glad she was happy.

Sometimes children have imaginary friends and say things that don't make much sense to adults. I thought Molly was having one of those experiences and I didn't think much about it. It was unusual for Molly to say things like this, as she possessed a down-to-earth personality and generally did not make things up like some kids do. I told Cheryl about it over breakfast and left it there.

Later that morning, Cheryl went to the post office with Molly to get the mail. On the way, Molly again mentioned Mary in the hospital room. Cheryl had not heard what Molly had said earlier. She asked her if she meant the little Mary statue that Katie had with her in the hospital bed. Molly said, "No, Mama, not the little Mary, big Mary." This was the first time Cheryl heard firsthand any of Molly's comments about Mary.

Cheryl told me about it when she got home, so I asked Molly about her seeing Mary in the hospital room again. Again, she said, "I saw big Mary, not little Mary, in the hospital room with Katie and she had her arm around Mama." Cheryl was still skeptical about it, thinking maybe Molly was making it up, but I don't think a two-year-old would do that uncoached. Neither one of us saw anything unusual in the hospital room during the few times when Molly was there to visit Katie.

In the day's mail there was a letter from my old friend Susan, a lady whom I had not spoken to or thought about for more than twenty years. I went to elementary school with her two sons, but she and the father of the boys had divorced and she moved to the West Coast years ago. Once in a while I saw the boys but I hadn't seen her for many years.

I opened the envelope and as I read the note inside, I was transfixed by her story. The letter expressed her condolences for our loss and told a story I had never heard. When she lived in California, Susan wrote, before she ever moved to our little town, she and her husband had lost a child who was four years old. She wrote that she was sure her little girl was playing with Katie and taking her around heaven and introducing her to all the angels and saints. Then came the line that floored me: "I am sure Katie and Elizabeth are getting along fine."

Cards and letters poured into the house. We received more than six hundred cards, many from people we had not heard from in years, most with a note and sometimes a check. One card was from a contractor friend of mine. There was no note, just his name: Scott. I loved it. There was a letter from the president of the finance company who held the note on one of my bucket loaders. He sent me a check to cover the payments for six months, which paid off the balance. Considering that it was a multi-billion-dollar international finance company, with tens of thousands of employees and millions of customers worldwide, it was a most remarkable and impactful gesture on his part.

Our friends and neighbors established an account at the bank where people could send donations. I am self-employed, so when I don't work, I don't get paid. It was through the generosity of our friends that we were able to survive financially during this time. We couldn't respond with thank-you notes. We were still overwhelmed.

In November the volunteer fire department held a pancake breakfast to benefit our family. They raised more than four thousand dollars in five hours, which they unselfishly gave to us as a donation. The money covered our house payment and bought groceries for a long time. Recovering from the death of one's child is a lengthy process. It was several months before I could safely go back to work.

One day in early November, we came home from some errand to find a tri-axle dump truck backed up to our woodshed. One of our neighbors had arrived while we were gone with a full load of cut and split firewood. We heat mostly with wood, and I had not had time to cut any while Katie was sick. He asked me if it was the right size for our stove, and I told him it was a little big but would do just fine. He said he would be back to help me stack it. The next day, to our great surprise, he brought yet another load, and I looked out to see a bunch of people swarming around the woodshed with my wood splitter running. There were five people splitting and stacking the wood in the woodshed. He wouldn't take any money for the wood, no one would consider taking any money for labor, and thus, six cords of wood were delivered, split, and stacked for us. We were ready for winter, thanks once again to the generosity of our neighbors. It was a huge help. And it came at a time when we really needed it.

We received a generous check from a man in Oregon whom we had never met. He was a friend of Cheryl's sister Debbie's boyfriend, Tim, and he wanted to contribute, though he had never met us or Katie. The generosity of this man and his wife ensured we would make it through the winter. Without these contributions, the loss of Katie would been compounded by financial difficulties. I don't know what we would have done without them. We are deeply thankful for the generosity extended to us in our hour of need.

About this time the medical bills started to arrive. Though we had good health insurance, it didn't cover all of the expenses. The total cost of Katie's three weeks in the PICU came to more than one million dollars. The helicopter ride alone was fifteen thousand dollars. Our insurance covered just over seven hundred thousand, leaving a bill of two hundred seventy-six thousand to pay. I just put it in the file. Later we got a notice that the hospital found the funds to cover it from a private donor. I was never sure if they just wrote it off or not, but we didn't get any more bills. We were able to pay the smaller medical bills that were not covered by insurance with the money people donated to us.

Late in the month we went to a granite monument shop to pick out a headstone. It was a small shop that I had done business with years ago. I liked the guy who ran it. We picked out a standard granite headstone and a flat stone with Katie's name on it.

After we completed our business with the monument company, we drove over to the next town to get some lunch. Before lunch, we stopped at the big box hardware store on the way. As we were leaving the store, I spied an elderly man with a limp walking along the driveway, headed out of the parking lot.

I stopped and asked him if he needed a ride somewhere. He readily accepted and climbed in the back of our little Toyota, almost as if he were expecting us. I asked him, "What are you doing walking around here, and where do you want to go?" His answer was cryptic: "I am just here checking up on you guys." I asked, "What do you mean?" His answer was, "I just wanted to see how you guys are making out. You can drop me off in the next shopping plaza if you don't mind."

I guessed this hitchhiker's age at seventy-four or more. He was a jovial fellow who presented himself as just a regular guy. When we came back from lunch an hour later, he was walking back to the big box store, so I pulled over to ask if we could give him a ride back. He told me no, he was all set, but thank you for the ride earlier. "I got what I came for," he said, though he was not carrying anything. It was a strange occurrence. Was he a messenger sent from On High to check on us? We don't know.

While we were at lunch, Dr. Connor called to ask how we were doing and if everything was okay with us. I was surprised that he called, now more than a month after Katie died, but I told him we were managing things. It speaks to the quality of care that the Boston hospital extends to the families of their patients.

CHAPTER 12

Winter of Our Discontent

That fall, winter came to stay before Thanksgiving, on November 20, with twenty inches of snow. It never stopped snowing until April. My brother Chris was the town road agent and I worked for him plowing snow on the town roads. I never liked plowing snow. One is at the mercy of the weather and must go to work when it calls. Often this is late at night and for long hours, in the worst of weather conditions. After working twenty hours behind the steering wheel of a snowplow, it takes a day or two to get back on schedule. This winter was unforgiving. It snowed about every three days, with a substantial accumulation each time. It turned out to be the second snowiest winter on record up to that time. We fought a big fight to keep the roads open and the snow pushed back with a wing, a special snowplow attached to the side of a plow truck, all the while preparing for the next storm to cudgel us.

I didn't have much time to think about things during the winter after Katie died. I suppose it was good to stay busy and well occupied. There were times, though, as I drove around in the truck plowing snow, when my thoughts turned to my little girl and her conspicuous absence from our life. These were perhaps the hardest times, because her loss was so recent. I thought about her all the time, wondering what went wrong, wondering if I had done something wrong or missed some small clue that might have saved her life. The fact was that she was gone, and I had to keep going, for Molly, for Cheryl, and ultimately, for myself.

Many friends called to check on our welfare. Xander and her sister, Ashley, were both attorneys in the Washington, DC, area and worked long hours. They would sometimes call me late at night. Receiving a call from them while out plowing went a long way toward cheering me up during those dark days.

There was one time during that winter when I distinctly felt Katie's presence. I was pushing back the snowbanks with my bucket loader on a narrow stretch of back road. I was all alone about nine o'clock at night, when I was sure I could feel her with me in the cab. She loved to ride with me in the machine and though it was crowded, I always made room for her. She wasn't there, but I was sure I felt her presence. This happened again later in the spring, when I was working on a project in the yard, building a cover over my dug well.

If I was outside, Katie had to be with me to help, no matter what I was doing. There was plenty for her to do, picking up pieces of wood or gathering nails. She loved it. That spring day as I was working, I suddenly had the feeling that she was right behind me. It startled me and I turned around, expecting to see her there, like so many times before. She was not there, not in bodily form anyway. Though I thought about her all the time, during these two incidents, I was focused on the task at hand, and not the memory of her. I was alone both times and I still wonder if my Katie girl was sneaking up on me and trying to surprise me the way she used to do.

At times like that I wondered if my mind was going, but I was otherwise functioning well and working hard every day. I didn't think I was depressed at the time, but looking back on it, I guess I was. Cheryl was down for months afterward but she was holding things together. She had received an extended leave of absence from her job through the end of her contract, which expired in April, eight months after she was notified it would not be renewed. This allowed her to stay home and recover. I kept in close touch with her during that time. She didn't like to talk about it that much, but I pressed her, looking for signs of serious problems. There were none, but we shared a mutual feeling of our tragic loss. Some studies show an increased divorce rate among couples who have lost a child, but other studies show a rate that is below average. Divorce never entered our minds. We became much closer during that time and neither one of us could imagine leaving the other at a time like that, or ever.

It was about this time when Cheryl reminded me of a dream she had had last summer, about a month before Katie became sick. In the dream she saw herself at a funeral, sitting in a chair holding Molly in her lap. It wasn't clear whose funeral it was, but the decedent was a child. She didn't see me in the dream but she was sure it wasn't my funeral. She'd put it out of her mind and never told me about it until now, afraid to believe it might be one of her children.

Molly was too young to understand and still made us laugh every day. Her stories about seeing Katie with angel wings continued through the winter, but became further apart as time grew on. We were careful not to say too much to her about Katie's death. We didn't hide it or gloss it over, but neither did we dwell on it in front of her. We tried to do a few fun family things on days that I didn't plow snow, but we couldn't go far, in case another big storm arrived to smother us. After Katie's death, nothing seemed to ease the pain. Time was the only thing that really helped.

January brought the news that Cheryl was pregnant. We were excited to think that Molly would have a sibling again. If the dates were right and the ultrasounds were right, the anticipated birth date would be in late September or early October. This was later refined to September 24, around the time Katie got sick the previous year.

In February we went to Boston to meet with Katie's doctors and go over the autopsy report. There was nothing particularly revealing. The doctors took time out of their hectic and demanding schedules to go over every detail and answer our questions. The one question they could not answer was why it happened. The official cause of her death listed three factors: cardiopulmonary failure, necrotizing pneumonia, and sepsis. While reading the report I noted that some of the laboratory examinations done on the tissue samples were conducted on her birthday, October 31.

We never did find out how she contracted the MRSA. What we do know is that two nasal swabs were taken at the first hospital, both of which tested negative for MRSA. She was swabbed again three hours later in Boston, twenty-three minutes after her admission, and tested positive for abundant amounts of MRSA. The germ has a rapid doubling rate, between twenty-eight and thirty-two minutes. Even at such a rapid rate of reproduction, we can't account for the difference between the initial test and the later one.

The negative predictive value of nasal swab tests for MRSA is very high, 99.2 percent accurate. The high predictability rate of the science would tell us that she acquired it sometime after she was tested the first two times. But Katie was already in acute respiratory distress when I brought her to Concord hospital. Four hours later she was bleeding so profusely that she coded, and should have died that night. Wherever she found it, it was already too late by the time I brought her to the hospital. The first test had to be a false negative. It wouldn't have mattered anyway.

The doctor who captured her on the first night told me that the damage to her lungs was similar to that found in victims of poison gas attacks—massive and widespread injury throughout both lungs. The autopsy report confirmed it. Where did she get the germ, and how, and when? Her doctors think her sickness might have been related to her immune system and how her body reacted. We don't know.

In March I started to write about our experience. It was difficult. Each day I would try to write something about it, to create the framework of what happened while it was still relatively fresh in my mind. The idea was to have a record of the event for Molly and for my eleven-year-old niece, and also for other family members and close friends who might want to know the whole story. Soon after I started writing I became infused with some kind of inspiration. I was able to write the majority of this story in eight days, in the evening after Molly and Cheryl went to bed.

I saved all the hundreds of letters and emails we received, to put them in a family album for Molly and other family members. I requested copies of Katie's medical records from her pediatrician and from the hospital in Boston. The request form asked what the records would be used for, and perhaps alerted the legal department that a lawsuit might be coming. The hospital sent the full record and did not charge me. It was three hundred pages long. The record was a dry chronicle of which medications and in what dosage they were given at which time. It was only a clinical record, but it helped me with the timetable of what happened and when, and helped lend some order to the writing of this story. I also recovered my cell phone log from that period. I thought it would help me to be able to document the events as they unfolded at the time in order.

Two people were encouraging and helpful to me at the time. One was Dr. Connor in Boston, who kept in touch and humored me by responding to my long and rambling emails. He told me to keep writing, to get it all down, and to publish it someday. One day I met with him in his office at the hospital to help me organize the manuscript. He took time to tell me stories of things he had seen happen in families after the loss of a child, and assured us there was nothing we had done wrong as parents. He told me that many people who write books about the severe illness or loss of a child have difficulty "getting it right." I wanted to do my best to get it right. I hope I did.

The other person was my eighty-year-old cousin, Tom Connors, in Scottsdale, Arizona. He heard about Katie's death while he was vacationing in Mexico, from the cable news networks. He was deeply upset by Katie's death and we corresponded frequently on many subjects. He had been battling cancer, but he found the time and energy to write me at a time when we needed positive people in our lives. Tom coached me to spend as much time as I could with Cheryl and to keep communication open with each other. Almost every day, he sent us a joke about our shared Irish heritage. Some of them were hilarious, playing on ethnocentric stereotypes. He was able to make us laugh when we didn't have much to laugh about. He died a few years later and I miss him.

In April it stopped snowing. We went to Washington, DC, to see the cherry blossoms and visit some museums. Molly loved the dinosaurs at the Smithsonian. It was good to get out of town for a while after such an awful winter. The warm air and bright sunshine brought us relief. We stayed with Xander's sister, Ashley, and enjoyed the city and her company.

When we came home it was back to business, but it was still not the same without Katie. There were days when I simply did not feel like working. Some days I went to work, and some days I stayed home. One of my friends asked me how we were doing. I told him we had good days, we had bad days, and we had very bad days, and we didn't get to pick what kind of day it would be when we woke up in the morning. We had to take it as it came and deal with it the best way we could for that day.

Katie's headstone was delivered in May. The owner of the shop moved his schedule around to be able to deliver it for Memorial Day, a huge effort on his part that we appreciate to this day. Because it was from a different shop than the one normally used in town, it had a different look than the other stones around it. It was a little wider than tall, which gave it a rather imposing, classic look. We liked it a lot. I poured the foundation for it, took my time, and got it just right. Later in the spring my friend with a landscaping business, Jon, delivered a load of loam, and I landscaped around it and planted new grass seed. The grass came in well, looked beautiful and lush; in that little country cemetery, the site looks idyllic. Sometimes I would drive by the cemetery on the way home, walk over to the grave, and check on the progress of the grass that was growing so nicely. I didn't do it every day, but it was refreshing to visit it every now and then and drink in the scenery.

On Memorial Day, the hospital in Boston held a ceremony to recognize the families who had lost children. We were invited to attend, and though Cheryl didn't feel up to going, being five months pregnant, I went down to see what it was all about. I met two friends from Boston there who had recently become engaged. They had visited Katie in the hospital room, and became quite emotional at the time. It was an emotional time, and they were still upset about our loss. (Later, after marriage and children and moving to the West Coast, the husband attained a doctoral degree, and his wife attended law school and ran for Congress twice, but didn't get elected.) The hospital did it right, with lots of flowers, a lady playing a giant harp, and sweet, soothing music, poetry, and songs to console a heavy heart. Each attendee was to choose a flower from a massive pail, proceed to the stage, deposit the flower in another large vase, and exit the stage. It felt to me like a graduation ceremony and I could almost hear the phrase "Welcome to alumni" as I left the stage.

CHAPTER 13

Glorious Summer

As the summer progressed Cheryl's pregnancy developed without complications. We went to the beach whenever we could get away. It rained almost every weekend. Starting in mid-June and going through July, it rained part of every day for six weeks. For a building contractor working outside, it was extremely frustrating, and some of my projects were delayed. I took a few beach days during the week if it wasn't raining, and squeezed in the work on the weekends to make up for it.

In August we had my friend Liam and his wife Marie over for a cookout. Liam had been my lawyer for years but got tired of making all that money and doing no work, and took a job as a government prosecutor. When dinner was over and we were lounging about laughing about politics, the phone rang. The caller identified herself as an investigative reporter from a Boston newspaper. She said she wanted to write a feature story about Katie and the germ that took her life. She was interested in highlighting the dangerous nature of MRSA, and said it was a timely subject matter. I knew from the caller ID that she had called several times before, but didn't leave a message. My future brother-in-law Tim in Southie had identified her to me several weeks before, since she had been pestering him, too. If nothing else, this lady was persistent, bothering us ten months after Katie's passing. I told her I would think about it and call her back.

While I was talking to her, Liam overheard me ask about the Boston newspaper the reporter worked for. That was all it took for his radar to flip into hyper-drive, and when I hung up, we had a spirited discourse on the press and newspaper reporters in general. I hadn't laughed that hard in months. I thought about it for a while, called the reporter back, and agreed to meet her. We agreed to meet at the Irish pub that I like to frequent, the one I went to with Katie, on the next weekend.

I did some research on her writing and she sent me copies of some articles she had published. What troubled me was the tone of her writing, the tone of a squinty-eyed conspiracy theorist, one who knew that those she wrote about were hiding something. Trying to keep an open mind, and recognizing that I was but a rude provincial, I met her at the pub on Sunday afternoon.

She presented herself well, poised and intelligent. She was cool and clever, perhaps too clever, not at all like the nitwits at the local newspaper. The problem was the tack she wanted to take with the article. Her idea focused more on the role of politics and public policy and how it affected the medical community and medicine in general, and not so much on the medical part. She wanted to use Katie's case as part of a larger story, or something like that, whereas I wanted Katie's case to be *the* story. I am sure she would have done a good job, but I wanted to present Katie's story to the world in a different way than she did. I just didn't want to work with her.

When we were done negotiating and started talking casually, she said she couldn't believe we didn't sue the Boston hospital. Surprised at her suggestion, I asked her why. She replied, "Well, your little girl was alive when she went in, and was dead when she came out. They killed her. You could get a huge settlement." I was stunned, and I was incensed. I didn't let it show, but that comment ended the interview and any chance of future cooperation. My mind was swirling, but I kept my cool.

After all they had done for Katie and for us, to think that we would turn around and sue the hospital to get money did not sit well with me. I was there with my Katie from the very beginning, from start to finish, twenty-one terrible days and nights. The doctors and nurses all rotated in and out on shifts, and different days brought different staff members. I saw what they went through. I watched every medication being given, I saw them resuscitate her four times, I watched them literally fighting to save her life. I attended every bedside meeting that was conducted. I saw the look in their eyes and on their faces. We experienced the deep generosity extended to us as a family in our most urgent time of need, by a caring staff who knew what we needed before we did. They killed her? Sue them? This reporter had it all wrong, and so do people who think like her. We parted amicably and left the pub, and I never heard from her again.

New Baby

When September came Cheryl was hot and uncomfortable and ready to have the baby. At four in the morning on the twenty-third, she announced it was time, got up, and started getting ready. I called my sister, Heidi, to come down to stay with Molly, and we rushed to the hospital. Her contractions were five minutes apart and I was concerned that we wouldn't make it to the hospital in time. I had a bag beside the bed with supplies to do a roadside delivery and I threw it in the backseat as we left. When we arrived at the hospital her contractions stopped. They kept us until noon and then sent us home.

Cheryl had intermittent contractions all day. My sister went home and waited. We ate supper and Cheryl again announced it was time. The contractions were back, five minutes apart. Heidi came back and we headed to the hospital again, checking in at seven thirty. We were assigned to a room and the signs were evident that this was not another false alarm. The doctor was called, we prepared ourselves, and Cheryl started having sharp labor pains at ten. The pain increased; the doctor examined her and said, "Okay, push!" The first time didn't work, but on the second push, after just fifteen minutes in labor, Kelly Ann arrived with a splash, at 10:15 p.m. on September 23. It was exactly one year to the day, and almost to the hour, that my Katie girl was admitted to the hospital in Boston.

A few days later we were back home when the church secretary, Claire, called, wanting to know all about the baby and how we were doing. She told me that because of the Christmas season approaching, there were only two dates available for baptism before St. Valentine's Day. One was in January, and the other was October 12. I was stunned. I said, "Okay, put us down for the twelfth." I then asked her if she knew what day that was. Her silence told me something must have registered with her, but it was too late. It was the day that Katie had died. She reacted immediately, falling all over herself with apologies and offers to change the date and work it in somewhere else. I said no, we would take that day and enjoy it. This was now the third baptism that was a bit atypical. And we now had two uplifting anniversaries to celebrate on the two sad ones, one year apart.

Kelly Ann brought with her all the things we had forgotten about little babies. Things like sleepless nights, endless laundry, diapers, and exhaustion. We were glad to have her, and at such a time. She was young for a baptism, only three weeks old, but we wanted to get it done, before some other crazy event happened to complicate matters. To think that we could do it on the anniversary of Katie's death was appealing to us. If I could stick my finger in the eye of the devil, I wanted to do it any way I could. I continue to wonder about the matches of the dates of Kelly's birth and baptism. I don't think they are coincidental.

Kelly's arrival heralded the true beginning of our path to healing. It was mostly because we had no time to think about anything else except her, and Molly. As she grew and developed, our attentions turned to the future, and her presence brought us much joy. Without recognizing it, we were forgetting about the bad times, as those memories were pushed out of our minds with good memories of Kelly and Molly.

It is a wonder to me to see the different personality traits of children when they are still babies, traits that are present from the time they are born. Katie was quiet at first and then became wild and rambunctious. Some mornings we would be awakened early to the sound of moving furniture. Three-year-old Katie was rearranging the furniture in her room, to make it better, as she would say. Molly was always quiet and content to be alone and play by herself. When Molly was two, on Easter Sunday, we did an egg hunt in the house for the kids. After the girls had collected all the plastic eggs and gathered all the candy, Molly disappeared with the basket of empty egg halves. A few minutes later, I went into the kitchen to find that she had taken the egg halves and placed them over the diamonds in the pattern on the vinyl floor. The entire floor was covered, with the eggs placed precisely over the diamonds. She was proud of her work and had done it all by herself.

Kelly was a screamer from the start, making it loud and clear when she wanted attention, which was most of the time. She kept us busy, focused on the immediate tasks of tending to an infant and helped, or rather, forced us to move on with our lives.

Katie's teachers at the preschool ordered a granite bench in her memory. It was supposed to be top secret, but I found out about it and asked if I could contribute in some way. They told me that the teachers had already paid for it and I was not to worry. As it happened, the bench was delivered to the school on the day before her birthday, one more strange occurrence. We received the call too late in the day to be present for the delivery, but Molly and I went down the next day, a Saturday, Katie's birthday, to see it. Her name is engraved on the top, a long-lasting memorial to our little girl.

CHAPTER 14

John and Cheryl

When Katie died, Cheryl and I were in a state of shock. The empty chair at the kitchen table was a deafeningly silent reminder of our loss and drove it home every night. We thought all along that she would somehow pull through. People were praying for her all across the country, in churches and prayer groups of all denominations. My mother broke her rosary beads by praying on them so often. Our church had special Masses for Katie and Father Ray asked everyone to pray for her and for us. While she was sick, I had even contacted a healing priest in the Boston area for special prayers. In our case those prayers were not answered. We believe there is an important reason why they were not, but the reason has not yet been revealed.

One of the groups of people praying for her was a contemplative prayer group in the North Attleboro area who were holding a twenty-four-hour prayer vigil. None of the members knew us or Katie, but the wife of one of the members knew Cheryl's mother, Ann. At precisely the minute of her death, 12:59 a.m. on Friday, October 12, this member experienced something from outside the natural world. He reported seeing a bright light fill the church while a figure appeared to those assembled. The figure was bathed in light and had radiant beams of light arranged behind her head, exactly as we see in the iconography of Eastern Orthodox and other similar religious paintings and icons. He said there was no doubt that it was Katie, and she delivered a message of peace and contentment, that all was well and the members could all go home. She was safe. He too felt the presence of a mature and liberated soul. He didn't talk about it until four months later, when he told my mother-in-law. When she told me, I called him and interviewed him. He said it was still frightening for him to think about but that we should be assured that Katie was all set.

Some of our friends asked us if we were going to counseling. Neither Cheryl nor I thought we could benefit from it. Katie was gone. We had to accept it and move on, or die ourselves. It came down to that. When Cheryl told her doctor that she thought she might be depressed, the doctor told her, "Your child has just died. Of course you are depressed." She offered prescription medications, but Cheryl didn't take them. I got a prescription to help me sleep while Katie was still in the hospital, but I took only two. They didn't work. An old friend invited me to attend a meeting of a support group for parents who had lost a child. Though I had known him for decades, I didn't know he had lost two sons, years before I was born. I thought about going to the group, but at the time I didn't think I was ready to talk about our loss. Cheryl and I stayed close to each other, to Molly, and later, to Kelly, and that was the best counseling either one of us could receive.

It is hard to articulate what we went through. One of my professor friends described it as ineffable, unable to be described. Cheryl told her mother on the day after Katie died that she felt a physical pain in her heart. She thought that was where the term "heartache" came from. I found that Cheryl was easily upset by talking about it, so after a while I limited talking about the queries that were constantly on my mind. We did talk about it, and a lot of other things, but there were no answers to our questions. It is easier now but it never goes away. The sense of loss is enormous. It feels as though a part of us has died. One of the books I read on surviving the loss of a child accurately stated that the timeline of our lives has been reset, bifurcated into two sections. One section contains everything that happened before the loss, and the other everything that happened after the loss. It's true.

We have the other children and we must give them all the things that children need, including a set of parents who are holding things together. In my private thoughts Katie is there all the time, laughing and ripping it up the way she always did.

Our entire community felt Katie's loss. In our small, rural town, everybody knows everybody else, and neighbors help neighbors. As late as eight months after she died, friends whom I hadn't seen or talked to since the event would see me at a job site or at the store or the dump. They would stop their farm tractors or big trucks and come over, hug me, and not let go. Most of the time, these burly, grown men were crying. It was powerful stuff.

We are not the first family in history to lose a child. It is only in our time, the time of our generation, that the death of a child is thought of as unexpected. I was talking to a doctor friend recently who remarked again on how unusual and rare Katie's case was. It was shocking to the medical community because, in the era of modern medicine, losing a child is rare. I have stayed in touch with many of Katie's doctors, and every once in a while, during our correspondence, one of them will opine on the unusual nature of her case, all these years later.

In the cemetery where Katie is buried there is a row of gravestones near the middle erected by the Nathaniel Huntoon family in the mid-1800s. Mr. Huntoon is buried on the end, the last of the family members interred there, in 1873, at age seventy-nine. A reading of the stones to the left of his tells a tale of heartbreak and horror.

He buried seven children, a grandchild, and his wife before he died, starting in 1827. Some of the children were two and three years old, some in their twenties and thirties. Some died within days or weeks of each other in the winter, and his grandson died three years after his mother. Her date of death is two days after the grandson's birth in December, and she probably died from complications of childbirth. Some died on the same date, years apart. How this man endured such a family tragedy is a source of inspiration to me. We lost one child and were completely unhelmed. This man lost seven, at all ages, and a grandson and his wife, over many years, and yet he endured. *The History of Salisbury* by John Dearborn, MD, published in 1884, tells us that Mr. Huntoon was a selectman and a justice of the peace during this time. Somehow, he found the strength to not just go on, but to serve his town at the same time, giving of his energy when it must have threatened to abandon him, as it did us, for many months. Dr. John Kepper, the town historian at the time, once told me that half of the gravestones in the cemeteries in my town are children aged ten and younger.

In the time of my father, the loss of a child happened far more often than it does today. He lost a four-month-old brother in 1933 to a condition that is easily cured today. Penicillin, the polio vaccine, and many other medical breakthroughs occurred after my father was born. Mortality statistics from the Centers for Disease Control and Prevention for the last seventy-five years show us that mortality rates for children ages one to four have declined 94 percent since 1935. Specifically, pneumonia caused by staphylococcus aureus in children aged one to four occurred only forty-five times in the fifteen years from 1999 through 2014. At the time of Katie's illness, there were only six cases of MRSA pneumonia in children on record anywhere in the world. It was extremely rare.

It's a different world today but even now, children die, and often. The difference is the prevailing and sometimes erroneous idea that modern medicine is invincible, that it can cure all ills and that children don't die. Medicine can work wonders, but we are still learning about the human body and its reaction to disease. There is much to discover.

There were some positive aspects to Katie's course. At least it was quick and it was relatively clean, and not "slow and obscene," to echo the words of Australian singer and songwriter Eric Bogle's "No Man's Land." We knew exactly where she was during the entire time. It could have been far more perverse. She could have been run over in our driveway by one of us, or hit by a car in a parking lot. She could have wandered off in the woods and died from exposure, or fallen down an abandoned well. She could have been kidnapped and raped, left in a ditch to die, and found a month or a year later, or maybe never found. She could have drowned in our pool or at the beach. The list goes on. One of my friends said, when I told him how thankful I was that it was quick, agreed with me. He said, "You're right. She could still be there."

One of the lessons I learned from the loss of Katie is that life is precious and brief. I remember watching former President George H. W. Bush being interviewed on television about the loss of his daughter when she was very young. I remember his words clearly: "Life is fragile." And so it is. A tragic loss like ours helps us to distill that which is important in life, and that which is not. Life is too short to fight over the minutiae.

When Kelly was eight months old, Cheryl decided to pursue a second advanced degree. She couldn't find a job as a biologist, and she had always wanted to study engineering. We decided that she should go for it, and she enrolled at the University of New Hampshire to pursue a second master's, this time in civil engineering.

The decision for her to go back to school meant that I would have to stay home with an eight-month-old and a three-year-old, as the cost of daycare was prohibitive. There was no work for me to do anyway at that time, due to a downturn in the economy. New Hampshire lost 95 percent of the jobs in the construction industry that year. It was a big load for me, functioning essentially as a single parent for twelve hours per day and more, and we became poor. The good part was that I was able to spend time with my girls and watch them grow and develop. Not every parent, especially fathers, gets that opportunity. Eventually, Cheryl graduated and found a job as an environmental engineer, while I stayed home and tended to the children. I sold most of my heavy equipment, discharged my employees, downsized the business, and worked part time.

On a warm spring day several years after Katie died, while Molly was in school, I was at home pushing Kelly, who was two and half years old, on the swing in the yard. Suddenly, in mid-swing, she looked over her shoulder, jumped off the seat, and started shouting, "Hi, Katie!" She ran toward the garden waving and shouting, saying, "Look, Daddy, it's Katie! Hi, Katie! And she's with Granny. At least I think it's Granny." This went on for five minutes and took me by surprise. I couldn't see anything, but Kelly could. Kelly is not an actress; she is a well-grounded person. In her mind Katie was there and Kelly recognized her, though she had never met her.

I called Cheryl at work and asked her to call her mother to see if she was okay. When her mother answered the phone and Cheryl told her the story, she started crying. She told Cheryl that she had just finished her afternoon devotions and rosary, and ended with a prayer asking for a sign that Katie was in heaven. As soon as she closed the prayer book, the phone rang. Here was the sign that she had asked for, delivered immediately upon asking for it. I thought maybe Kelly had seen a vision of Cheryl's grandmother walking with Katie, since Cheryl's mother and grandmother look more like sisters, and twin sisters at that, than mother and daughter. She died in 1988.

CHAPTER 15

The Lilac Project

On Memorial Day, a year and a half after Katie's death, we went to the cemetery to plant some purple petunias on her grave. Purple was Katie's favorite color and we always found purple flowers to plant for her. As I surveyed the area around the cemetery, it occurred to me that though it was located in a beautiful country setting, the immediate area seemed rather bare. There were no permanent plantings of flowers anywhere. The closest thing to flowers was the presence of some widely scattered multiflora roses along the perimeter.

Those roses were planted by one of our neighbors, Howard Moxley, to create a barrier around the cemetery and to add some beauty to the grounds. Howard had donated a piece of land to expand the cemetery in the late 1950s and wanted to improve the looks of the fence line. One evening in 1963, when he didn't come home for supper, his wife, Iva, called my father, who went down to the cemetery and found him dead from a heart attack. He had been digging fence post holes for the new fence being installed and planting the roses. It was too much for him in the summer heat. That was the last time any planting had been done at the cemetery.

I thought about what kind of flowers we could plant that would grow in the poor soil and harsh climate of New Hampshire. We needed flowers that would not present a maintenance problem for the mowing of the cemeteries, and that would be in bloom around Memorial Day. And they should be purple. The idea struck me like a thunderbolt: lilacs. I was inspired that day, standing at Katie's graveside, to start the Katie Bentley Lilac Project. Since it was inspired, I cannot claim credit for it. I am convinced it was Katie's idea. She tried to tell me a few weeks after she died with those lilacs that bloomed unexpectedly in the fall, but I didn't get it. It took me a year and a half and even then, she had to hit me over the head.

New Hampshire has had a love affair with lilacs for more than two hundred and fifty years. The oldest documented lilacs in North America are located in Portsmouth, New Hampshire, at the Wentworth-Coolidge Mansion and date from at least 1750. New Hampshire is the only state in the country that has the purple lilac as the state flower. In 1939, Governor Murphy declared Arbor Day to also be Lilac Day in New Hampshire. Between 1945 and 2003, the University of New Hampshire introduced ten new lilac cultivated varieties, or cultivars, to the nursery trade, including "Miss Kim," the most widely planted lilac in the United States, and one of the best-selling lilacs worldwide. New Hampshire has lilac bragging rights.

At first, I envisioned a hedge of purple lilacs running all around the fence line. But I took a lesson from the multiflora roses planted a half-century before, and realized that would be too much. The roses were a maintenance problem, growing six feet a year, finding their way into the mowed areas, creating a tangled mess of sharp thorns and ugly, dead canes. A lilac hedge would overpower the old cemetery and block the view of the field and hills behind it. A few lilacs planted far apart would enhance the beauty of, but not overwhelm, the pastoral scene.

There were obstacles to implementing my idea. The first was the policy of the cemetery commission, which stated that no permanent plantings could be installed in any town cemetery. As one who had mowed the cemeteries for years, I knew this was a good idea and a sound policy. Permanent plantings interfere with the mowing and maintenance of the grass. My idea was to leave plenty of space around each lilac plant, so the lawn mowers could keep them in check over the years. Planting them along the perimeter would also prevent the maintenance person from having to take extra care mowing around them in the cemetery proper, where space is tight and the headstones already present obstacles to a speedy finish.

There was also the problem of the lilacs themselves. I didn't know a lot about them or where to buy them in quantity. Lilacs at the retail nurseries were expensive. Still, the idea was there and wouldn't go away, so I did my homework.

The first hurdle was to approach the cemetery commission. I had served on the first cemetery commission when it was established in the early 1990s, and Cheryl had served on the same board in the early 2000s, so we knew how things worked. I went to a meeting with them and explained what I wanted to do, and to my surprise, they thought it was a good idea. The cemeteries could use some improvement, they thought, and the lilac project was a low-impact way to do it.

The next hurdle was the money. I talked to my certified public accountant and started the process of creating and registering a non-profit entity with the state and the Internal Revenue Service. We started it with some of the money we had left from the donations we received after Katie died.

I made a poster and put it around town with Katie's picture on it and a story about what we were doing. I asked for small donations from the townspeople. Money started to come in, by five- and ten-dollar checks. Some people gave a lot more, including my cousin Tom Connors from Scottsdale. It was his and his wife Mary's donation that really got things off the ground. We raised more money than we needed to plant the lilacs at Katie's cemetery, so we expanded the plan to include the other cemeteries in town.

I found a nursery in Massachusetts to supply the lilacs. They had more than twenty thousand plants of various sizes, representing more than three hundred cultivars. The weather was hot and dry that summer, so we delayed planting until the fall. The first batch of lilacs was planted at Katie's cemetery in mid-September.

The teachers at Katie's school heard about it and expressed interest in planting some lilacs. I contacted the director of facilities at the school district, an old friend who was two years ahead of me in high school. He loved the idea. We found spots in the traffic islands where no problems with snow removal or traffic lines-of-sight would be encountered, and planted a few next to the buildings. We acquired a mature "Marechal Foch" lilac to plant next to Katie's memorial bench. The school librarian was having a mural painted on the vaulted ceiling in the library, showcasing the elementary school and the grounds. She had the artist paint lilacs into the mural, lilacs that we had not planted yet. She helped create the landscape plan for the school with the mural.

Planting the lilacs at the cemeteries in town created a lot of interest. It was a popular event and caught everyone's attention. The town office went so far as to dedicate page 2 in the annual report to Katie's memory and the lilac project. Included was a color picture of Katie and of a lilac named "Royal Purple," the first lilac we ever planted, near the front gate at her cemetery. It was the first time that color pictures had ever been included in a town report.

In May, one of my friends in the governor's office asked if the governor would issue an official proclamation in support of our work planting the state flower. The governor remembered us and readily agreed to do it. On June 25, we were invited to the New Hampshire State House to meet with His Excellency and have our photograph taken with him as he presented us with the proclamation. It was a huge shot in the arm for the Katie Bentley Lilac Project. It announced to the world that it wasn't just us who thought we had a good idea.

In the fall we were featured on the cover of the alumni magazine at one of my alma maters. It wasn't *Rolling Stone*, but it was the cover, and we were on it, posing with the governor of New Hampshire. The Katie Bentley Lilac Project had arrived. We are now represented in ten states by more than three thousand lilacs in hundreds of locations, where the flowers can be enjoyed by all.

We planted four hundred lilacs throughout the school district. Interest in lilacs was high. Fourth graders study the history of New Hampshire, so I created a short presentation on the history of lilacs in our state for them. I made up some bookmarks with pictures of lilacs representing the seven colors of the Wister Code. The Wister Code, developed by the late John Wister in the 1940s and 1950s, is a general way of classifying lilacs by color.

I also compiled a booklet with color pictures and lilac history and facts to distribute to the students. The best part of the presentation, the part the students love the most, is a small lilac in a pot for them to take home and plant. The lilac project gets bigger every year and is becoming a lot of work. We provided lilacs to four hundred students last year. The excitement of the fourth graders makes it worth it. This is how the next generation of lilac lovers is created. It underscores the unique history of the lilac in New Hampshire in a hands-on way that the kids will remember forever.

My work with lilacs brought me to the International Lilac Society. It is a group dedicated to lilacs that boasts members from all over the world. I served two terms on the board of directors, and was recently elected treasurer of the organization. I encourage the reader to visit their website, and if lilacs are something one loves or wants to learn more about, to join as a member. The website is www.internationallilacsociety.org.

We had been dabbling in charity work before Katie ever got sick. Our primary goal then was to provide winter gear and diapers for underprivileged children in New Hampshire. The director of the daycare that Katie and Molly attended once told me that some of the children came back to daycare in the morning wearing the same diaper they wore when they went home. She would discreetly mark the back of the diaper with a pen, which was how she figured it out. We bought several boxes with our own money and gave them to the daycare center. Sometimes we would buy winter coats for the kids who didn't have one.

It was apparent now, however, that we needed to incorporate if we were to become serious about our charitable efforts. We incorporated as the Katie Bentley Memorial Charity, d/b/a Katie Bentley Lilac Project. As a registered charitable entity, we would be better able to receive donations from donors. Buying boxes of diapers to give away or receiving leftover coats for free from a big box store and holding them in our garage for six months was one thing. Before we could accept any money, we had to be registered with the state and federal government and assemble a board of directors to oversee operations. It took twenty-two months to receive our tax-exempt status from the IRS, but the state application was easy and completed in less than a week. We now have a board of professionals in their respective fields, all with the same commitment to supporting those less fortunate. We don't have a lot of funding, but we do a lot with what we receive. Last year, we were able to donate more than six thousand dollars' worth of clothing, diapers, and winter coats to the daycare center and the school district. A few years ago, I received the Champion for Children Award. It is given by the New Hampshire School Administrators Association as recognition for service to children. I won the regional award and the statewide award, and received two plaques and a donation to the charity as a prize.

I wanted to make the lilac project universal. Though the project was rooted in our personal tragedy and named after my Katie girl, I wanted it to reflect a positive ending to that tragedy. I encouraged people to join the Katie Bentley Lilac Project simply by planting a lilac in the name of their own lost loved one, or just because they love lilacs. That way it could apply to anyone who experienced the grief of loss of a loved one, or to anyone who shared our love of lilacs. Every year when the lilac bloomed in the dooryard or garden, one would be reminded that life does go on. The poised form of the lilac flower thyrse with its pleasing aroma would bring dignity and hope with the renewal of spring.

A couple of years after Katie died, on Halloween, her birthday, a Bloomerang lilac planted near our deck spontaneously burst into bloom—not in the spring, but in the fall, after several hard frosts. I took it as a sign that Katie approved of our lilac project.

A granite monument in a cemetery is stately, but cold. A lilac flower in one's yard planted in memory of someone brings a warm and joyous feeling. That is what the Katie Bentley Lilac Project is all about. The lilac project that carries her name continues to grow, carrying with it the message of hope and renewal. Every time I see a lilac in bloom, I think of her not in death, but as she was in life: beautiful, precocious, and full of love. The lilac project is Katie's legacy to the world; not a bad accomplishment for a four-year-old girl from New Hampshire.

CHAPTER 16

Pneumonia, Again

On Katie's birthday, Halloween night, four years after she died, Molly began to get sick with a cough and fever. It was snowing hard. An early-season blizzard had arrived in New Hampshire. I didn't like the course she was exhibiting, so I decided to take her to the hospital. I feared I might be overreacting because of Katie's sickness, but it was time to have her checked.

We went to the same hospital as I did with Katie, in Concord. The staff on duty that night consisted of almost the same team who had treated Katie four years earlier. One of her teachers, the librarian at her preschool who painted lilacs on the ceiling, was wearing her other hat as a paramedic that night. Even the doctor who sent us to Boston on the helicopter was there. When they learned that a six-year-old girl in respiratory distress with Katie's last name was in the ED, they pushed the panic button. Unknown to me at the time, Katie's course had caused them to implement a review of how such cases were handled, and they were much more aggressive than in the past.

We were ushered into the back in a hurry, with nurses and doctors running from all directions to her bedside. Curtains were pulled back so hard they almost came off the track, trash cans were kicked out of the way, and the chairs in the room were thrown into the hallway and pushed aside, to make room for the number of people crowding into her triage room.

I began to have horrifying flashbacks. I eased myself out of the room, just like before, and I was stunned to witness a near repeat of what I had seen in Boston. Lined up outside of her room was a group of eighteen people, some with crash carts, some carrying little baskets with different meds, one pushing a portable X-ray machine, all of them silent, waiting to be called to perform their specialized role.

Leading the charge, dressed in her scrubs with a stethoscope around her neck and a walkie-talkie in her hand, was the librarian turned paramedic. There was no doubt about who was in command of the triage area that night. She was giving directions, talking into the radio, helping people move their carts, directing people where to go and where to wait. Katie's doctor, Geoff, was at Molly's bedside, ordering tests and evaluating Molly's condition, speaking and responding to questions in that same direct, measured tone I had heard before in Boston. I couldn't believe what I was witnessing. Though sick, Molly was composed and seemed to be enjoying the attention. I was terrified.

Because of the blizzard, I knew there would be no chopper ride that night. We were on our own. The outcome of Molly's course would be determined right there in that room. We were trapped.

The team diagnosed Molly with pneumonia, but not bacterial pneumonia, the kind that Katie had. This was a rare occurrence: a parent relieved to hear that his child had viral pneumonia. That year pneumonia was common in our area. This was the third time Molly had contracted pneumonia in the last two years, so the team decided to admit her and monitor her progress for a few days. They weren't taking any chances.

Twenty-four inches of snow fell with that storm. I had to leave Molly there overnight so I could go home and plow the driveway, but we went to see her early the next morning. After that, one of us was able to stay with her most of the time. It started out much like what we went through with Katie, but this time it was short and with a much better outcome. Molly was discharged two days later. I think Katie had a hand in how things ended.

Twelve years after Katie passed, when Kelly was eleven years old, Kelly woke up with abdominal pain. I took her to the same ED at Concord Hospital at eight thirty in the morning. The team determined that she had a kidney infection, and the machinery began to move. They admitted her and started massive doses of antibiotics to get the fever and infection under control. Her fever kept going up, and by ten at night, was at 104.5, dangerously high. Half an hour later it was at 104.7, and the medical team started to panic. The doctor told us that if it went to 105, they were calling a helicopter and sending us to Boston.

I sent a text message to Dr. Connor, outlining what was going on with Kelly. He called me back immediately, at 11:45, almost midnight, and asked me some questions about Kelly's course. He said if I wanted, he would send a chopper to pick her up right then, get her into the PICU, and in his words, "See if we can save her."

Luckily, by midnight, fifteen minutes later, her fever started to abate, and came down rapidly. By one in the morning, it was down to 102, and everybody breathed a sigh of relief. It had been close. The attending physician told me we "dodged a cannonball, not just a bullet." She told me there is an eighteen-hour window from the onset of kidney infection symptoms until death occurs. We barely made it under the wire. The fever went away, Kelly came home, and she slept soundly upstairs. We had a follow-up with her pediatrician a few days later, and he fine-tuned the dosage on her meds. What a difference a day or two makes.

This was the third time, once for each of the girls, where we were in a life-threatening situation, either requiring evacuation by chopper or on deck to be taken out. It's no wonder my hair is white now. A friend of mine told me that he thought I had developed a "thousand-yard stare" after Katie died. I can't see it.

CHAPTER 17

How We Coped

Because of their sicknesses, and the loss of Katie, Cheryl and I look at the world differently now. We take a longer view of events, and make time to stop and enjoy simple things. We have a small spruce tree on our lawn, a wedding gift from my brother, and we hang Christmas lights on it every year. Because we had so much snow during the winter after Katie died, all the branches were heavily covered, obscuring the needles. A dull light was still visible through the snow, and it appeared as if the whole tree was aglow with some kind of inner energy. We had never seen that before, and we haven't seen it since. During the summer after Katie died, my great-grandmother's rosebush bloomed better than we had seen it in decades. Lilac bushes in full bloom hold a special meaning for us now. It is that kind of simple beauty that we take time to notice and enjoy.

The worry about the children never goes away. It's always there, ready to spring into our consciousness, an unknown malevolent force lurking just beyond the wire in the bushes. Our story is not new or unique. Many children die each year the world over, thousands every day. Who knows what the child may have meant to the world and to history had they lived to offer their own special contribution? Stalin wrote, "The death of one man is a tragedy; the death of one million is a statistic." Yet each one of those deaths studied individually is still a tragedy.

Cheryl and I consider ourselves lucky and blessed beyond measure to have had access to the services of the hospital in Boston. In much of the world those services are just not available. We tried, and the hospital staff tried, and tried hard, but we lost. Katie has moved on from this world to the next. She lives on in our memories.

What do I take away from the loss of our child?

I learned that our locus of control is not what we think it is. We can make plans, and most of the time, well-laid plans will come to fruition. Sometimes, though, they don't. When that happens, the only control we have is how we react and respond to sudden changes. Behaving with dignity and grace during times of unexpected upheaval is rooted in acceptance of the fact that we are not always in control of events around us. We have to bob and weave and adapt quickly.

I learned that the choices we make early in life have a lasting impact. Choosing the right partner for marriage is important. Actively practicing and participating in one's religious faith is important. Getting as much education as one can stand is important. And it's important to develop and maintain good relationships in life. What would we have done without the help we received from our friends and neighbors? It would have made it so much harder.

All these things give us a foundation upon which to build our lives and raise a family, the four legs of a stool, so to speak. When trouble presents itself, we possess the arms and shields to do battle. Life is not always easy or fair, and the more help we have to face our troubles, the easier it is to defeat them, corporeal or spiritual.

In his book *Man's Search for Meaning*, Austrian psychiatrist and Holocaust survivor Viktor Frankl wrote that mankind yearns to find meaning in life. When faced with extreme adversity, those who have identified a meaning in their lives do better than those who have not. Belief and hope in the future is closely tied to and dependent upon one's understanding and embracing of their inner self, the spiritual self.

I decided that I was the only person who was going to be able to help me get over the challenge faced by Katie's death, and it would come from my inner self. We were good parents, Katie was healthy, she received the best medical care in the world. Still, she died. It was a crushing blow, with no explanation. Dr. Connor called it bad luck. My philosopher friend Ken called it an asteroid—no way to prepare for it, no way to defend against it. The loss simply had to be experienced and endured—and within that loss, find the meaning. We could only overcome it from the inside. My philosopher friend from South Korea once referred to this inner strength as *chi*. It's a universal concept.

Some people have asked me what advice I would give to a family who has lost a child. I'm never sure what to say. Each case is different, no two families are alike. What we did was to pull in our horns and focus on just us for a while. I had been trying to extricate myself from a lot of my activities, especially politics, for years. Cheryl and I were always ready to volunteer for any number of things. She was active in her quilt guild, served on a few town boards, and went to PTA meetings. I had been a volunteer for different town activities for decades, from the cemetery board to cooking chickens at the barbecue on Old Home Day. I couldn't do as much as I used to after the girls were born, and after we lost Katie, I couldn't do any of it for quite some time.

The headwinds we faced were enormous. In two weeks that September, Cheryl lost her job of fifteen years, my brother-in-law was diagnosed with leukemia, and Katie got sick. Any one of these events places a burden on a family. Though the debacle with the news coverage about Katie's death was short lived, it added to the stress we were experiencing. How many more droplets of misery in the pan would it take to tip the scales and make one of us lose our sanity? Turning off the phone and the television, closing the gate on my driveway, reducing all external stimuli, and trying to counsel each other was all we could do. We stayed close to each other and did as many family activities with Molly as we could. We avoided people for the most part. Nobody knew what to say. Everyone was uneasy and uncomfortable, even our closest friends.

It's important not to make any major decisions in the period immediately following such a tragedy. We had enough money to get by, so we tried to relax and absorb and process the event. It took us months before we enjoyed any kind of normal lifestyle again. We still ran the blood drives with the hospital, but that was only two or three times a year. Cheryl's parents did most of the work, though we would go down and help out when we could. I went to a few support group meetings in the spring after she died, public events that friends had invited me to attend, with hundreds of people, but I wasn't attracted to the environment. Things were too busy there, and I needed solitude.

Seeking that solitude, one day in the summer following Katie's death, I went back to a secret fishing hole I hadn't visited since I was a teenager. It was still the same: verdant, secluded, and full of trout. I kept a few, and released the others. That part of my life hadn't changed. It was refreshing therapy.

Our experience with Katie's death revealed to us that there is indeed a heaven, just as we have been taught to believe. The stories that came to us from Molly and others were too frequent and too unusual to be manufactured, especially by a two-and-a-half-year-old child. The incidents we witnessed were too many, too disconnected from each other, and too complex to be simply coincidences or fantasies. Some of my atheist friends dismiss them all as imagination or accident. They don't believe. They have no faith. At a minimum, they should review Pascal's wager. Even Huckleberry Finn said his prayers, just in case. One of my college professors offered a Freudian explanation, that during times of extreme duress, the mind creates situations that reinforce and affirm previously held beliefs. That theory didn't fit with the stories we heard from other people.

With a profound and unexpected loss like ours comes the risk of becoming angry with The Almighty. We never did. We have faith, and for us, we believe we have confirmation of that faith. The reader must make his or her own decision.

The End

Do not fear, I am with you;
Do not be anxious:
I am your God.
I will strengthen you,
I will help you,
I will uphold you with My
Victorious right hand.

—Isaiah 41:10

If the reader would like to support our ongoing charity or lilac-planting efforts, a donation in any amount may be mailed to Katie Bentley Memorial Charity, PO Box 269, Salisbury, NH 03268. All donations are tax-deductible to the extent allowed by law. The Katie Bentley Memorial Charity is a 501(c)(3) tax-exempt organization. www.katiebentleylilacproject.com

Appendix

Katie's Funeral Brochure

In Loving Memory of Catherine Ann Bentley 10/31/2002–10/12/2007

Katie was born to John and Cheryl Bentley on Halloween morning, at 4:35 a.m., 2002, in Concord Hospital. She was only 7 pounds, 7 ounces, but she grew rapidly, and did not walk until she was twenty-two months old. Katie was a big girl for her age, and very stout. Her strong personality developed early on, and she became something of a character at a young age. She would often introduce herself to complete strangers in grocery stores and at different functions, always making people laugh with her forward and friendly demeanor.

Katie was very strong willed and a wild daredevil, always going down the tallest slide or jumping from the highest diving board, and wanting to swing ever higher on the swing set. She loved music and she loved to dance, breaking out in perfect rhythm to whatever genre happened to be airing at the time the spirit moved her. At parties and functions, she stole the show, and was never shy about working the crowd or ripping it up on the dance floor.

Katie attended preschool and absolutely loved her teachers and classmates, looking forward to and talking about class each day. She was warm and caring, often comforting children her own age who were hurt or crying. Of all the fun she had, she loved swimming most of all, and her family made it a point to take Katie and her sister Molly swimming at every opportunity.

Katie was especially close to her paternal grandmother, Ruthann Bentley, nicknamed Tanny, her cousin, Annie Stetson, and maternal grandmother, Ann Allen. She was perhaps closest to her little sister, Molly, always watching over her beloved playmate and partner in crime.

Katie was a beautiful, vibrant, loving child who touched the lives of everyone she met, and will always be remembered in the same loving way by those who knew her. God bless her in heaven.

About the Author

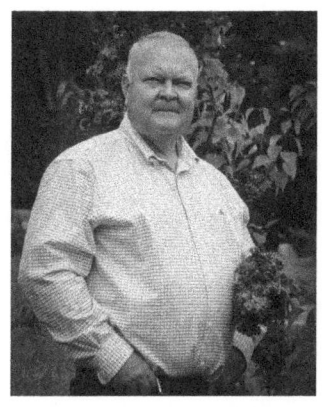

John Bentley, a New Hampshire native, grew up in a small town surrounded by nature, stone walls, extended family, and good neighbors. Over the years, he has worn many hats, working as an automobile mechanic, sawmill laborer, farmhand, excavation contractor, carpenter, machinist, purchasing agent, and college administrator. For almost forty years, he has also served as the cemetery sexton in his hometown. John holds a bachelor's degree in business administration from Southern New Hampshire University.

In his spare time, John operates a small nonprofit charity that provides winter clothing to underprivileged children. He serves as treasurer of the International Lilac Society and enjoys growing lilacs and ornamental plants, vegetable gardening, woodworking, restoring horse-drawn vehicles, and fly fishing with his daughters using flies they tie together at the kitchen table during winter. A voracious reader and amateur historian, he is actively involved in several local historical societies. John lives with his wife and two daughters on a small farm near a brook, down a long dirt road, deep in the woods.